Beyond Pain

The Study Companion

By

Thomas Moshiri MD

Printed in the United States of America

ISBN 13: 9-781-4414-7795-8

ISBN 10: 1-4414-7795-0

Every effort has been exerted to assure the completeness and accuracy of the information contained within this book. However, in view of ongoing research, and the constant flow of information relating to the practice of medicine, the reader is urged to exert professional responsibility when applying this information in a particular situation or clinical circumstance. The author, editors, or the publisher are not responsible for errors or omissions or for any negative consequences from the application of the information contained within this book. Medicine is an ever changing field and no warranty is expressed or implied with respect to the currency, completeness, or the accuracy of the contents of this publication.

For further information or to contact the author please visit:

www.BeyondTheBoards.com

Preface

I'm really happy that you have decided to purchase this book! Not because I'm going to receive a commission from the sale, but because you are genuinely serious about learning and mastering the information in *Beyond Pain: A Comprehensive Pain Board Review*. Although it is not necessary to own both copies in order to prepare for your pain board certification exam, I find that the two books complement each other in such a way that they enhance the learning process significantly.

This study guide is a highly focused summary of the major ideas found in the board review book. By boiling chapters down to their essence, this study guide will give you the framework to build on as you learn new facts. Each chapter of this book correlates directly with the same chapter in the board review book in order to assist the reader in correlating the information obtained from both resources easily and quickly.

What you will find at BeyondTheBoards.com and specifically in *Beyond Pain: The Study Companion* is a complete and thorough review of the material you need to know in order to achieve top notch knowledge in the field of Pain Management. My intention is to completely immerse you in the field and keep you *continuously updated* so that you can achieve superior knowledge that can be utilized during your clinical career. In addition, my goal is not only to help you prepare for what lays ahead, but to provide you with the knowledge needed to continue to succeed throughout your career and beyond.

It is clear that medicine is as much a business as it is an art. Yet, we receive no education in Asset Protection, Tax Reduction, and Wealth Preservation during our medical training. While my intention is to help you prepare for your board certification exam, I also intend on helping you learn more about business and finance as it relates to physicians. So, study hard, use the resources available to you here and once you've passed the boards as I'm sure you will with persistence and dedication, come back and visit us at BeyondTheBoards.com for further education.

Finally, if there are any comments or recommendations for improvement with respect to this board study material, if there are any mistakes that should be corrected, or if any changes have occurred of which I am not aware, please help me and your colleagues stay updated by contacting me through my website.

I would like to dedicate this book to my lovely and caring wife Rien who has continuously supported me through this endeavor and has motivated me to shift out of "park" and into "drive"!

Table of Contents

READ THIS SECTION!

How to Use This Book

Beyond Pain: The Study Companion is designed to test your knowledge and solidify the information learned in the Board Review Book. It is designed to work in synchrony with the Board Review Book and as such no answers are provided in this study companion. This book correlates each chapter with the same chapter found in Beyond Pain's Board Review Book and utilizes multiple testing formats in order to drive the information home and make it stay there!

The test formats utilized include fill in the blanks which will focus your attention on gaps in your knowledge, matching questions which will help you build associations between related terms and facts, true or false statements which will force you to solidify your core knowledge, and finally short paragraph answers which will challenge you to consolidate your learning and to master key concepts from the text. Multiple choice questions are rarely used because that specific testing format is mostly passive and does not promote active learning. It is easy to fool yourself about how much you are remembering as you read and choose the "best" answer. The testing format employed in this *Study Companion* will help you actively process information, so that you can recall and apply what you know more quickly and effectively.

The Study Plan

Begin each day by reading a chapter of *Beyond Pain: A Comprehensive Board Review* and taking notes based on each section of the chapter. If you resort to highlighting, you may find yourself highlighting entire pages so I would refrain from that specific study technique. At the end of your study session, review your notes and then go back and review the contents of the chapter you read the day before. Now, open up *The Study Companion* and go through the corresponding chapter from the day before to test your knowledge. This gives you the chance to practice recalling facts from your reading, after you've closed the book. I would recommend that you review each Board Review Book chapter *at least* three times. There are 38 chapters in the review book, if you study one chapter per day, and review the book in its entirety three times, you will require approximately 120 days (that's four months!) so do not procrastinate. If you truly know all the material in this book, not only will you guarantee your ability to pass the board examination, you will also become a better physician. The study plan outlined above is not an easy one, but then again nothing worth having ever comes easy!

Anatomy of the Brain and the Cranial Nerves

1. Write the name of the structure and any associated Cranial Nerves in the image below:

Internal View of the Base of the Skull

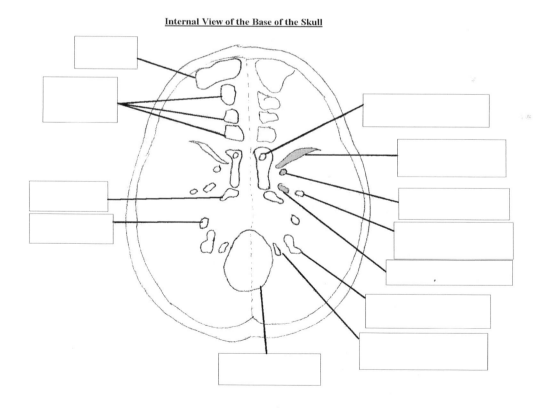

2. Review the Thalamus in *Beyond Pain* and fill in the blanks below:

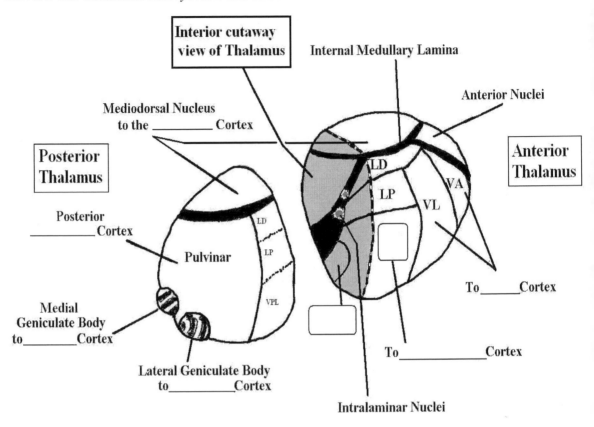

3. Where is CSF produced? Trace the path of CSF utilizing the following structures: Interventricular foramen of Monro, Aqueduct of Sylvius, foramen of Luschka, and foramen of Megendie.

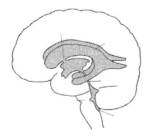

a. CSF bathes the spinal cord and is reabsorbed by spinal epidural veins into the general circulation.   **TRUE or FALSE**

4. There are two components to our perception of pain. These include the _____ component which relays information from the dorsal column to the limbic system. The other is the _____ pathway which relies on information exchange from the lateral thalamus to the somatosensory cortex.

5. The ascending spinal nociceptive pathways rely on the following neurotransmitters: (choose best answer)

    1. NE, GABA, TNF α, Calcitonin G related protein (CGRP)

    2. Substance P, Glutamate, CGRP, TNF α

    3. Serotonin, NE, Opiates, and GABA

    4. Substance P, Opiates, NE, Serotonin

    5. Serotonin, Glutamate, GABA, CGRP

6. All of the cells in the Spinothalamic tract project to the contralateral thalamus.   **TRUE or FALSE**

7. The axons of the Spinothalamic tract project only to the VPL, VPM, VPI, VL, and LP nuclei of the Thalamus.   **TRUE or FALSE**

8. The Spinothalamic tract helps to mediate the sensations of pain, cold, warmth and touch.   **TRUE or FALSE**

9. The Cervicothalamic tract arises from neurons in the lateral cervical nucleus. The cervical nucleus receives input from Laminae III and IV. The axons travel to the _____ side and ascend in the medial lemniscus of the brain stem to nuclei in the midbrain and to the VPL and VPM nuclei of the thalamus.

10. Most axons of the Spinomesencephalic tract originate from Laminae IV-VI as well as Laminae X and the ventral horn. Some of these neurons give off collaterals that end in the lateral thalamus. The axons project in the _____ anterolateral quadrant of the spinal cord to the Mesencephalic reticular formation and periaqueductal gray matter (PAG) and via the Spinobrachial tract to the Parabrachial nuclei.

11. The PAG is a synaptic location for descending inhibitory fibers.

TRUE or FALSE

12. The Spinoreticular tract is composed of axons from Laminae VII and VIII. These axons ascend in the _____ anterolateral quadrant of the spinal cord and terminate in the reticular formation of the Medulla.

13. The Spinohypothlamic tract is comprised of axons from Laminae I, V, and VIII. It projects directly to the _____ centers and is thought to activate what type of responses?

14. What is the role of the Postsynaptic Dorsal Column tract? What types of fibers innervate these axons?

15. There are a few descending inhibitory pathways which originate from the periventricular grey matter. What are the inhibitory neurotransmitters upon which these pathways rely on?

16. The Periaqueductal Gray (PAG) sends excitatory signals to the Locus Coeruleus (LC) in the Pons which in turn sends inhibitory signals to Laminae II, III, and IV in the dorsal columns. **TRUE or FALSE**

17. The cranial nerves responsible for carrying Parasympathetic fibers include CN-X, CN-IX, CN-V, and CN-II. **TRUE or FALSE**

18. The Trigeminal Ganglion is also referred to as the _____ Ganglion. It resides in _____ which contains CSF. This ganglion divides into three branches. The Ophthalmic branch exits via _____, the Maxillary branch exits the _____,and the Mandibular branch exits _____.

19. What are the contents of the Pterygopalatine fossa?

20. Match the cranial nerves to their function:

I- Olfactory _____

1. Motor to stylopharyngeus muscle, parasympathetic to parotid gland, visceral sensation from the carotid body, general sensation from posterior 1/3 of the tongue

II- Optic _____

2. Taste to anterior 2/3 of the tongue, parasympathetic supply to all glands of head except parotid

III- Oculomotor _____

3. Special sensory for balance, hearing

IV- Trochlear _____

4. Motor to pharynx and larynx, parasympathetic to all thoracic and abdominal viscera

V- Trigeminal _____

5. Motor to sternocleidomastoid and trapezius muscles

VI- Abducens _____

6. Special sensory smell

VII- Facial _____

7. Motor to lateral rectus

VIII- Vestibulocochlear _____

8. Motor to intrinsic and extrinsic muscles of tongue except the palatoglossus

IX- Glossopharyngeal _____

9. Special sensory vision

X- Vagus _____

10. Sensory from surface of head and neck to sinuses, meninges, and external tympanic membranes. Motor to muscles of mastication.

XI- Accessory _____

11. Motor to all extraocular muscles except superior oblique and lateral rectus (SO4-LR6)

XII- Hypoglossal _____

12. Motor to superior oblique muscle

21. Match the cranial nerve with the parasympathetic fibers it carries:

CN X (Vagus) _____

CN IX (Glossopharyngeal) _____

CN VII (Facial) _____

CN III (Oculomotor) _____

1. Pupil constriction, accommodation

2. Lacrimal gland, Mucosal glands of nose and palate, Submandibular and Sublingual glands

3. Parotid Gland

4. Heart, GI system

Anatomy of the Spine

1. Imaging considerations of the spine:

   a. MRI is good at looking at bone, while CT scans are good at looking at soft tissue.   **TRUE or FALSE**

   b. T1 weighted images are better for visualizing _____ which appear white on these type of images. T2 weighted images are better at visualizing _____ which appear white on these type of images.

   c. T1 images are good at looking at the bony structure of the vertebrae.

   TRUE or FALSE

   d. Under what circumstances would one utilize contrast?

   e. Myelography involves the injection of contrast into the intrathecal space. What are some of the reasons one would use this type of study?

f. Discography has multiple components including volumetric, manometric, radiographic, and pain provocation (concordant or discordant).

  i. Volumetric exam involves injecting contrast into a disk. The maximum volume that can be placed in a lumbar disk is _____, while a cervical disk can take _____.

  ii. Manometric evaluation involves transduction of pressures with increased disk volume and is a very objective study.

  TRUE or FALSE

  iii. What is concordant pain on discography and how is it different from discordant pain?

  iv. List at least three complications that may occur with discography. Is it useful to administer antibiotics with this procedure?

2. Anatomy of the Cervical spine:

   a. The lower cervical segments from C3-C7 consist of a 5 joint complex.
      This complex is composed of one _____, two
      _____, and two uncovertebral joints of
      _____.

   b. Fill in the blanks in the image below:

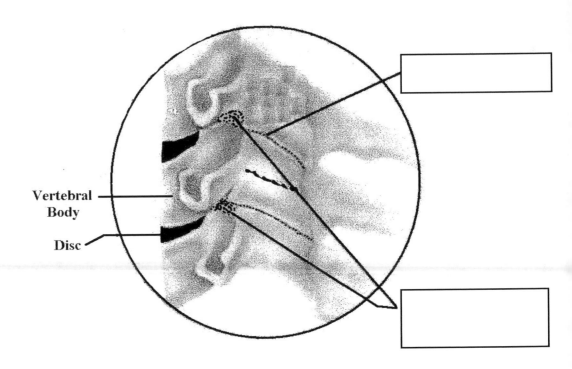

   c. In the cervical region the nerve roots exit below the given pedicle.
      Hence the C5 nerve root exits below the C5 pedicle.

                                                    TRUE or FALSE

d. To view cervical facets on x-ray, a lateral view should be obtained. If one wishes to view the foramen, an oblique view should be obtained. Is this any different in the lumbar region and if so how?

e. Where does the median nerve lie in an AP view of the cervical spine? How about in the lateral view?

f. In the cervical region, each particular facet is innervated by the median nerve from the current level, and the level above. In the Lumbar region, each facet is only innervated by the median nerve from the current level. **TRUE or FALSE**

3. Anatomy of the Lumbar spine:

   a. The lumbar region consists of a 5 joint complex. In the lumbar region there are two uncovertebral joints of Luschka, one intervertebral disc, and two facet joints. **TRUE or FALSE**

   b. If there is a disk herniation at L4-L5 which nerve root will most likely be affected?

      a. L3
      b. L4
      c. L5

c. What type of disk herniations are more common and why?

4. Abnormal anatomy of the spine:

  a. The disk is made up of two components: the Annulus fibrosis and the Nucleus pulposus. Which of the following characteristics best describes the intervertebral disk? (choose the best answer)

    1. The Annulus fibrosis consists of concentric lamellar rings around the disk, the outer 1/3 of which is innervated.

    2. The Nucleus pulposus is primarily composed of fat.

    3. The intervertebral disks are vascular structures.

    4. Vertebral endplates are susceptible to fractures which can disrupt the vascular supply and cause micro-hemorrhage.

  b. Internal disk disruption can be diagnosed by _____. This is a painful medical condition, and is the earliest form of DDD marked by disk dehydration, loss of disk height, subchondral marrow changes, and an annular fissure.

c. Utilizing the relative amount of extrusion of the disk circumference, what is the difference between a generalized disk bulge and a focal herniation?

d. A disk protrusion is the same as a herniation and an extrusion. The difference is the extent to which the disk bulges into the epidural space. Which of the following four statements is true?

    1. In an axial view, a disk protrusion has a larger y-axis span than x-axis extension.

    2. A herniation has a small extension on the x-axis and a greater extension on the y-axis (its extending into the epidural space more).

    3. A disk extrusion is simply a herniation that extends cranially and caudally. A disk extrusion is *not* in continuity with the disk.

    4. A disk sequestration is an extrusion where the segment is in continuity with the disk.

e. Extrusions and sequestrations will enhance with contrast which is another reason to obtain a contrast study when there is a mass in the lateral recess. **TRUE or FALSE**

f. Spinal Stenosis, Lateral Recess Stenosis

    i. Below are the three proposed etiologies of stenotic pain in an individual. Explain how each of these patients will present:

        1. Arterial insufficiency:

        2. Venous congestion:

        3. Compression:

    ii. Cervical spinal stenosis is associated with myelopathy whereas lumbar stenosis is not usually associated with myelopathy. Why?

iii. Indicate the motor neuron deficiency associated with each of the following signs:

Sign	Upper or Lower Motor Neuron
Weakness	
Fasciculation	
Up-going plantar response	
Atrophy	
Hyperreflexia	
Hyporeflexia	
Spasticity	
Flaccidity	

5. Pathologic conditions of the spine:

   a. Vertebral bodies

      i. DISH syndrome (diffuse idiopathic skeletal hyperostosis)

         1. DISH syndrome is associated with pain and stiffness. It is non-radiating in nature. How is this disease diagnosed radiographically?

         2. How is this condition different from ankylosing spondylitis?

    ii. Ossification of the Posterior Longitudinal Ligament (PLL)

        1. This condition can coexist with DISH.

TRUE or FALSE

        2. It can lead to LE symptoms and eventual bladder dysfunction.   **TRUE or FALSE**

    iii. Ankylosing spondylitis is a spine calcification disorder. Calcification of the annulus and the ligaments gives rise to the term _____ which lacks flexibility and is susceptible to fractures.

b. Impingement upon spinal nerve roots

    i. Define and distinguish between *Radiculopathy, Radicular pain,* and *Radiculitis:*

c. Disorder of alignment

    i. Define the following five types of Spondylolisthesis:

        1. Dysplastic

2. Spondylo-lytic

3. Degenerative

4. Traumatic

5. Pathologic

    ii. How is the diagnosis of Spondylolisthesis made? Slippage greater than what distance would indicate an unstable spine requiring surgical intervention?

6. Spinal anatomy:
   a. The spine can be conceptually divided into three compartments; Anterior, Middle, and Posterior. The anterior compartment is innervated by _____. The middle compartment is innervated by _____ which make multiple connections at multiple levels of the spine. The posterior compartment is innervated by _____ of the dorsal ramus.

7. Treatment Paradigm:
   a. Considering the etiology, and the pathogenesis indicated below, fill in the possible treatments for each condition:

Etiology	Pathogenesis	Rx
Annular tear	Leak of mediators, altered mechanism	
Protrusion, Herniation	Leak of mediators, compression	
Facet and SI	Biomechanical	
Failed Back Sx	Multiple	

   b. Intradiscal Electrothermal Coagulation (IDET) can be used to cause contraction of collagen tissue, thermal denervation, and granulation tissue formation. Name at least three conditions which may warrant the use of this treatment technique:

   1.

   2.

   3.

Anatomy of Thorax and Abdomen

1. Thorax:

    a. What is Tietze syndrome?

    b. The Phrenic nerve innervates the peripheral diaphragm.

    TRUE or FALSE

    c. The mediastinal and the diaphragmatic pleura receive innervation from the Phrenic nerve.　**TRUE or FALSE**

    d. Describe how the convergence-projection theory explains referred pain.

2. Autonomic Nervous System:

a. The ANS as a whole is divided into a sympathetic and a parasympathetic system. **TRUE or FALSE**

b. The sympathetic system ranges from T2-L2. **TRUE or FALSE**

c. The sympathetic system is composed of short preganglionic and long postganglionic fibers. **TRUE or FALSE**

d. The parasympathetic system involves cranial nerves X, IX, VII, III (1973) and S2-S4. **TRUE or FALSE**

e. The parasympathetic system is composed of short preganglionic and long postganglionic fibers. **TRUE or FALSE**

f. The sympathetic ANS preganglionic fibers travel to a para-vertebral sympathetic chain ganglion via WHITE rami where they synapse and exit as GRAY rami, ascend/descend the sympathetic chain, or they travel further to a Pre-vertebral ganglion.

TRUE or FALSE

g. The prevertebral ganglion includes the Celiac ganglia, the Aortic plexus, the Superior Hypogastric plexus, and the Inferior Hypogastric plexus. **TRUE or FALSE**

h. The Splanchnic nerves are derived from T5-T12. **TRUE or FALSE**

i.   The Vagus nerve contains motor, somatic, visceral afferent and
     parasympathetic fibers.   **TRUE or FALSE**

j.   Sacral roots S2-S4 send long preganglionic fibers to the pelvic
     splanchnic nerves and onto the pelvic inferior Hypogastric plexus.

                                                       TRUE or FALSE

k.   The visceral afferent sensory system is a sympathetic system.

                                                       TRUE or FALSE

l.   Autonomic efferent centers in the spinal cord include: (fill in the
     blanks)

        1.   Head and Neck _____
        2.   Heart sympathetic _____
        3.   Thoracic sympathetic _____
        4.   Lungs sympathetic _____
        5.   Abdominal sympathetic _____
        6.   Pelvic parasympathetic _____

3. ANS pharmacology and its relevance to neurotransmitter release at various
    ganglions:

    a. In the SNS the preganglionic neurons release Ach onto _____
        receptors in the sympathetic chain ganglion. Postganglionic neurons
        then release Noradrenaline onto _____ receptors.

    b. In the PNS the postganglionic neurons release Ach which acts on
        _____ receptors.

Anatomy of Upper and Lower Extremities

1. Please fill in the blanks in the image of the Brachial Plexus below. Also state which muscles are innervated by each of the nerves tested:

<u>Brachial Plexus</u>

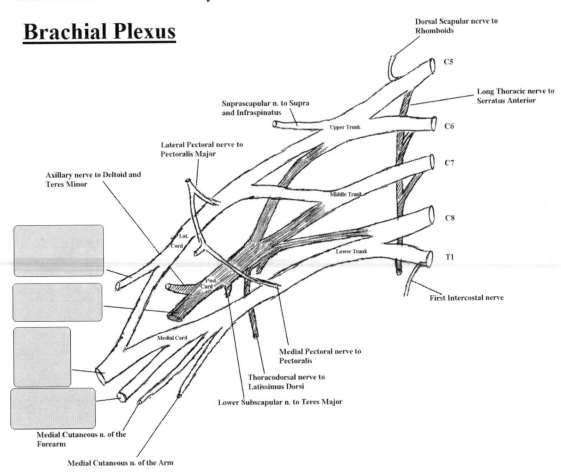

a. Match the motor, reflex, and sensory function for each nerve:

Nerve	Motor	Reflex	Sensation
C5	_____ Finger flexors, hand intrinsics	_____ Biceps reflex	_____ Medial forearm, med. Ant. Brach. Cutaneous nerve
C6	_____ Hand intrinsics	_____ Triceps reflex	_____ Medial Arm, med. Brach. Cutaneous nerve
C7	_____ Forearm pronation and supination, wrist extension and flexion.		_____ Index and Middle finger, dorsum of hand
C8	_____ Deltoid, Biceps	_____ Brachio-radialis reflex	_____ Lateral aspect of forearm, thumb, and index finger
T1	_____ Triceps extension, wrist flexion and extension, finger extension		_____ Lateral arm, Axillary nerve, deltoid numbness

b. Match the major peripheral nerve with its motor and sensory function:

Nerve	Motor	Sensation
a. Radial (C6-8)	_____ Deltoid	_____ Lateral arm,
b. Ulnar (C8-T1)	_____ Biceps	_____ Lateral forearm
c. Median (C6-8,T1)	_____ Wrist extension, thumb ext., triceps, brachialis, brachioradialis, supinator	_____ Distal ulnar aspect, little finger
d. Axillary	_____ Thumb pinch, opposition of thumb (ok sign), abduction of thumb, pronator	_____ Dorsal web spaces between thumb and index finger
e. Musculocutaneous	_____ Abduction, flexor hand muscles, little finger	_____ Distal radial aspect, index finger

c. What is Tinel's sign? What is Phalen's sign? Why are they used?

d. DeQuervain's syndrome occurs due to (choose the best answer):

    1. Inflammation of the abductor pollicis longus

    2. Inflammation of the abductor pollicis brevis

    3. Inflammation of the extensor pollicis brevis

    4. Inflammation of the extensor pollicis longus

    5. 1 and 3 are correct

    6. 2 and 4 are correct

    7. All are correct

2. Lower Extremity Anatomy:

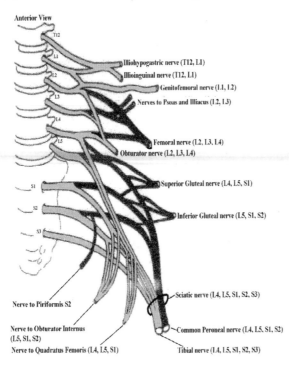

3. Review the lower extremity dermatomes:

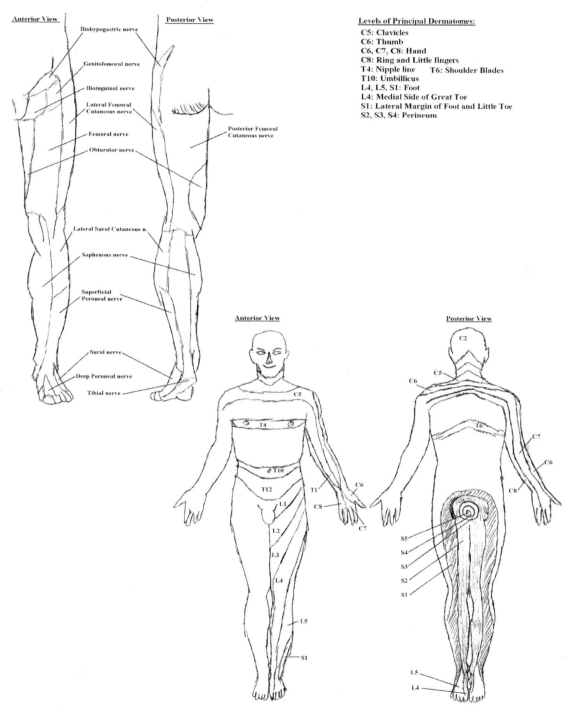

Levels of Principal Dermatomes:
C5: Clavicles
C6: Thumb
C6, C7, C8: Hand
C8: Ring and Little fingers
T4: Nipple line   T6: Shoulder Blades
T10: Umbillicus
L4, L5, S1: Foot
L4: Medial Side of Great Toe
S1: Lateral Margin of Foot and Little Toe
S2, S3, S4: Perineum

a. Foot drop occurs due to the compromise of which nerve root?

b. The Achilles reflex tests which nerve root function?

c. What is the "anal wink" sign? What does it demonstrate?

d. The Sciatic n. (L4-S3) innervates the hamstrings, muscles of the leg and foot, and it is sensory to the outer leg and the whole foot.

TRUE or FALSE

4. Match the major peripheral nerve with its motor, reflex, and sensory function:

Nerve	Motor	Reflex	Sensation
L4	_____ Extensor hallucis longus	_____ Achilles heel reflex	_____ Dorsum of the foot and lateral leg
L5	_____ Peroneus longus and brevis	_____ Knee reflex	_____ Lateral aspect of the ankle and foot
S1	_____ Tibialis anterior	_____ No reflex to check	_____ Medial aspect of foot

5. Fill in the blanks on the following pages, indicating the nerve(s) responsible for the indicated movement:

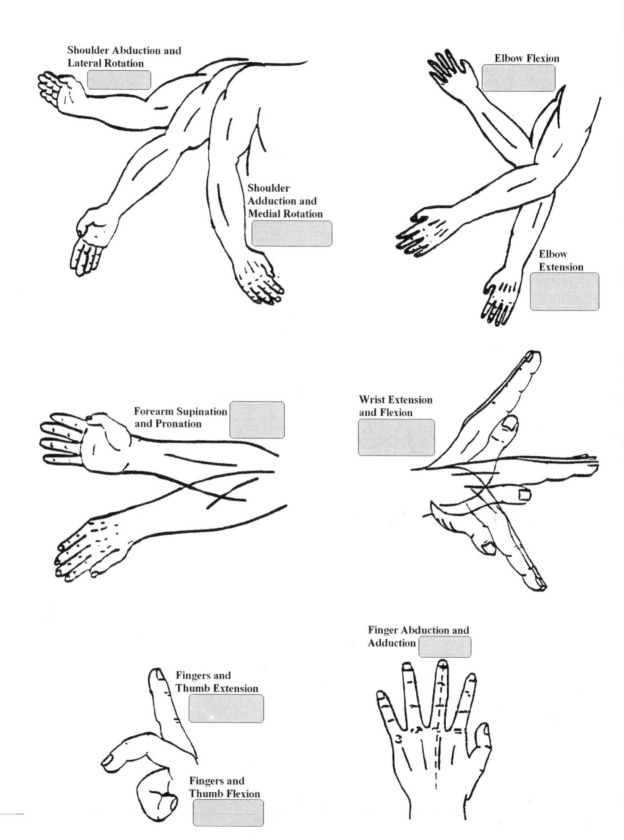

Shoulder Abduction and Lateral Rotation

Shoulder Adduction and Medial Rotation

Elbow Flexion

Elbow Extension

Forearm Supination and Pronation

Wrist Extension and Flexion

Fingers and Thumb Extension

Fingers and Thumb Flexion

Finger Abduction and Adduction

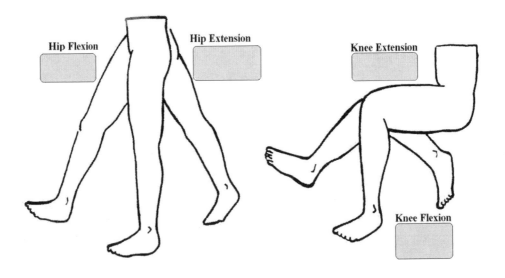

Hip Flexion

Hip Extension

Knee Extension

Knee Flexion

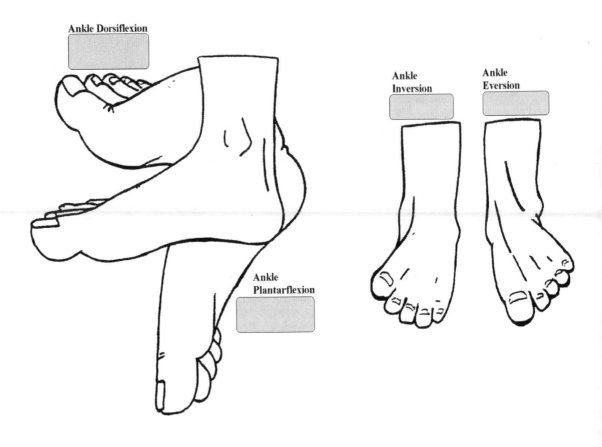

Ankle Dorsiflexion

Ankle Plantarflexion

Ankle Inversion

Ankle Eversion

Basic Biology of Pain Processing

1. Organizational anatomy of pain pathways:

   a. Match the axon type to the correct diameter, velocity, and effective stimulus:

Axon Class	Diameter (Micron)	Velocity (m/s)	Effective Stimulus
A-Beta	_____ 0.5-1.5	_____ (Group II) > 40	_____ High threshold thermal, mechanical, and chemical, FREE nerve endings
A-Delta	_____ 12-20	_____ (Group IV) < 2	_____ Low & High threshold mechanic or thermal
C	_____ 1-4	_____ (Group III) 10-40	_____ Low threshold mechanoreceptors, specialized nerve endings i.e. Pacinian Corpuscles

   b. C fibers are activated by a multitude of stimuli, hence they are referred to as "Polymodal" fibers.   **TRUE or FALSE**

   c. At the sensory terminal, all transduction proteins function through voltage sensitive sodium channels.   **TRUE or FALSE**

d. Transmitters that evoke post synaptic excitation in the dorsal root ganglion include: (choose the best answer)

    1. Substance P which binds to NK-1 receptors

    2. CGRP which binds to P2X receptors

    3. Glutamate which binds to NMDA receptors

    4. ATP which binds to AMPA receptors

    5. Choice 1 and 3 are correct

    6. I don't know, I'm really confused!

e. After activation, the initial depolarization of the nerve terminal is mediated by Glutamate which yields an acute transient depolarization followed by Substance P which yields a slow persistent depolarization.

TRUE or FALSE

f. Substantia Gelatinosa is associated with Rexed Laminae II, and A-Delta and C fibers.   **TRUE or FALSE**

g. Nucleus Proprius is associated with Rexed Laminae V, and A-Beta and C fibers.   **TRUE or FALSE**

h. Laminae V neurons receive a "convergence" of input from both the A-Beta, as well as the A-Delta, and C fibers. They are referred to as Wide Dynamic Range (WDR) neurons.   **TRUE or FALSE**

i. Different axons (i.e. Sympathetic afferents) converge onto WDR neurons; this convergence on a single spinal neuron gives rise to referred pain.   **TRUE or FALSE**

j. The WDR nuclei in Laminae V send signals via the contra lateral tracts to the thalamus (VPL) via the Spinothalamic tract or the Spinoreticulothalamic tract.   **TRUE or FALSE**

k. Describe the Spinoreticulothalamic tract. How is it different from the Spinothalamic tract?

2. Post Tissue Injury Processing:

a. After peripheral injury, numerous factors are released which have the ability to activate the nerve terminal. These products include 5-HT, Proteinases, Cytokines, Growth Factors, Bradykinin, Prostaglandins, K+, H+, Substance P, and CGRP.   **TRUE or FALSE**

b. Persistent cell depolarization by the inflammatory "soup" leads to nerve terminal sensitization so that any following stimulus yields a greater response.   **TRUE or FALSE**

c. "Windup" is the enhanced response of a WDR neuron in the face of a continuous C-fiber stimulus.   **TRUE or FALSE**

d. Repetitive C-fiber stimulation enhances the response characteristics of the WDR cell in such a way that for any given input you get an even greater output.   **TRUE or FALSE**

3. Mechanisms of dysfunction after nerve injury:

    a. After acute focal injury to a nerve axon, the proximal portion will begin to sprout a new axon. If contact between the proximal axon and the distal axon is not made, a cluster of free nerve endings result referred to as a _____.

    b. Sensory axons normally have no spontaneous afferent activity.

TRUE or FALSE

    c. Neuromas show increased activity in NaV channels, and an increased expression of neurotransmitter receptors leading to spontaneous afferent traffic and spontaneous dysesthesia.

TRUE or FALSE

    d. Nerve injury can lead to tactile allodynia secondary to: (choose the best answer)

        1. Increased dorsal horn excitability due to the activation of low threshold mechanoreceptor afferent neurons.

        2. Loss of dorsal horn GABA and Glycinergic neurons.

        3. A-Beta axons sprouting into Substantia Gelatinosa causing reorganization of dorsal horn connectivity.

        4. Post-ganglionic sympathetic axons sprouting onto a Neuroma or the DRG and activating those cells.

        5. Activation of both Astrocytes and Microglia.

        6. All of the above are true

        7. Some of the above are true (circle the correct ones)

        8. Um, I think I need to read this chapter again!

Cancer Pain

1. Cancer types and related questions:

   a. Pain can occur due to direct tissue invasion of the brain and meningeal stimulation. **TRUE or FALSE**

   b. Bone metastases are the most common type of cancer related pain. The thoracic vertebrae are the most common site of bone metastasis.

   TRUE or FALSE

   c. For any type of direct tumor invasion of nerve _____ provide excellent analgesia.

   d. Factors which predict whether breast cancer will metastasize include:

      1. Increased production of (PTHrP)
      2. Positive estrogen receptor
      3. The level of tumor differentiation
      4. Tumor response to Tamoxifen
      5. 1,2, and 3 are true
      6. 1 and 3 are true
      7. All are true

e. Lytic lesions have increased _____ activity. These kinds of lesions are most commonly seen in _____.

f. Sclerotic lesions have increased _____ activity; there is an increase in bone mass and decreased pathologic fractures. The incidence is greatest in _____ cancer which actually produces osteoblast stimulating factor.

g. Bone metastasis can occur due to:
   1. Hematogenous spread due to the presence of vertebral venous plexuses.
   2. Contiguous spread most common in Multiple Myeloma
   3. Lymphatic spread which is more common on the left side of the vertebra.
   4. Local extension via peri-organic fat
   5. None of the above
   6. Some of the above (Ooops, better go back & review!)

h. What are the characteristics of metastatic bone pain? Does this type of pain respond to NSAIDs?

i. What diagnostic tools are available to screen for bone metastasis? What are the advantages and the disadvantages of each?

j. X-ray is a poor screening tool but it is a good tool for _____ _____ because it is a lytic osteoclastic disease process.

k. Which type of scan is the "gold standard" for detecting tumor metastasis but is a poor choice for "cold" tumors?

l. List at least three treatments which are available for bone metastasis?

     1.

     2.

     3.

m. Multiple Myeloma (MM) is a tumor of plasma cells (Plasmacytoma). MM presents with classical _____ lesions on x-ray.

n. Clinical manifestations of MM include pathologic fractures, hypercalcemia, renal failure, cord compression, and hyper-viscosity syndrome.   **TRUE or FALSE**

o. Which of the following evaluation tools regarding MM is correct?
   1. Increased ESR
   2. Impaired coagulation due to inhibitors of clotting factors
   3. Impaired platelet function
   4. Monoclonal gammopathy
   5. Bence-Jones proteinuria on urine protein electrophoresis (UPEP)
   6. All of the above are correct

p. Prostate CA presents with osteoblastic bone lesions.

TRUE or FALSE

q. Prostate CA can metastasize to the long bones & vertebrae causing spinal cord compression and perineal pain. Visceral pain can also develop due to ureteral obstruction secondary to retroperitoneal lymph node extension. **TRUE or FALSE**

r. Breast CA most commonly metastasizes to _____, _____, _____, and _____.

s. If estrogen receptors are present and the tumor is well differentiated, the incidence of bone metastasis decreases. **TRUE or FALSE**

t. Analgesics have been shown to help when lymphedema occurs due to poor upper extremity lymph drainage after mastectomy.

TRUE or FALSE

u. Radiation Myelopathy is in essence a post radiation cord ischemia. It presents as a _____ Syndrome which is ipsilateral motor weakness and loss of vibration, and contralateral loss of pain and temperature.

v. If a single cranial nerve palsy is present the most common diagnosis is _____.

w. Unlike Oat Cell lung CA, Small Cell lung CA is sensitive to chemotherapy and radiation. **TRUE or FALSE**

x. Small Cell lung CA is typically centrally located on x-ray and presents with rapid growth and early metastasis.   **TRUE or FALSE**

y. Paraneoplastic syndromes are more common with Non-Small Cell lung cancer.   **TRUE or FALSE**

z. In contrast to the Oat Cell lung CA, which type of lung cancer is located peripherally on chest x-ray?

aa. Pancoast Tumor is characterized by:

    1. A subset of lung cancers that invade the apical chest wall.

    2. A tumor that lies outside the lung and invades the adjacent extrathoracic structures including the chest wall, nerve roots, lower trunks of the brachial plexus, sympathetic chain, stellate ganglion, ribs, and bone.

    3. Most commonly a squamous cell carcinomas or adenocarcinoma.

    4. Typically involving the Phrenic nerve, Long Thoracic nerve, or superior vena cava.

    5. All are true

    6. Some are true (circle the correct answers)

bb. Hypernephroma (Renal Cell CA) can present with paraneoplastic syndromes. What are these syndromes?

cc. Describe Carcinoid syndrome. What are the signs and symptoms of this syndrome? Which hormone is most commonly secreted?

2. Oncologic Emergencies:

   a. Hypercalcemia of Malignancy is the most common paraneoplastic syndrome.

      i. Humoral hypercalcemia is associated with which type of lung cancer?

      ii. Local Osteoclastic Hypercalcemia is associated with which type of cancers?

      iii. List at least three treatment options for Hypercalcemia:

         1.

         2.

         3.

b. Spinal Cord Compression can result in the loss of the "anal wink". The sensory level affected will be 2 levels below the compression.

TRUE or FALSE

c. An MRI can be helpful in distinguishing between infection, tumor, or the identification of a sequestered disk. **TRUE or FALSE**

d. Describe the presentation of patients with SVC Syndrome. Which diagnostic tool is most useful in discovering the primary tumor?

Central Pain States: Diagnosis and Management

1. Neuropathic pain can be due to a peripheral or central etiology:

    a. Identify and differentiate between CRPS I (formerly RSD) and CRPS II (formerly Causalgia).

    b. In peripheral pain, the time of onset coincides with the onset of a lesion or pathologic process whereas in central pain, there is a delayed onset of days to months.   **TRUE or FALSE**

    c. Central pain lesions are demonstrable by electrophysiological studies.

    TRUE or FALSE

    d. Analgesics always help peripheral and central pain symptoms.

    TRUE or FALSE

    e. Central pain can be abolished by nerve blocks and neurectomies.

    TRUE or FALSE

f.   Spinal cord lesions can induce central pain.

TRUE or FALSE

g.   Syringomyelia pain is usually experienced in the areas of dissociated sensory loss. The syrinx can be seen in _____ weighted images.

2.   Pathophysiology of central pain:

a.   Central pain is believed to be a result of increased neuronal activity and increased neuronal _____ along somatosensory pathways.

b.   It is believed that the fibers that travel via the lateral Spinothalamic tract are denervated and the feedback that modulates incoming impulses from the _____ fibers is over written.

c.   The dorsal column medial lemniscus does not have to be involved to elicit central pain.   **TRUE or FALSE**

d.   The A-beta fibers coming into the cord are interrupted; hence the _____ fibers are left un-inhibited. There is also inhibition of _____ allowing Glutamate and Substance P to go unchecked.

e.   There are three thalamic areas involved in the development of central pain and they are the _____, _____, and_____ nuclei.

f.   In a brainstem lesion, the same side of the body and the face are affected.   **TRUE or FALSE**

3. Spinal cord injury:

   a. Cord lesions present with thermal pain threshold abnormalities.

   TRUE or FALSE

   b. Deficits of dorsal column function (including touch, vibration, & position sense) are rarely seen in spinal cord lesions but common in supraspinal central pain.   **TRUE or FALSE**

   c. Describe the signs and symptoms of anterior spinal artery syndrome.

   d. Complete the table below which differentiates between the pain pattern of spinal stenosis and disc herniation:

	Disc Protrusion	Spinal Stenosis
Pain Pattern		
Response to conservative Tx	>90%	50%
Age at onset	30-50	>60
Radiography		
Myelography		
CT, MRI		

4. Multiple Sclerosis:

   a. In MS pain may be localized to the lower half of the body, one or both legs, or ipsilateral arm and leg.   **TRUE or FALSE**

b. Patients with Trigeminal Neuralgia below the age of 50-60 are unlikely to carry the diagnosis of MS. **TRUE or FALSE**

c. The first line drug for treatment of Trigeminal Neuralgia is

   _____.

d. MS pain is described as mostly burning, aching, and stabbing. Tonic seizures are seen. Pain is generally related to spasticity.

   TRUE or FALSE

e. What is Lhermitte's sign?

5. Post amputation, Phantom limb pain:
   a. How does the neuromatrix (Walzack) theory explain phantom pain?

6. Treatment of Central Pain:
   a. Please describe the first, second, and third line treatment options for central pain:
      i. First line:

      ii. Second line:

      iii. Third line:

Discectomy

1. If a disc herniation is in the paramedian location at L4-5, the nerve actually affected is that of _____.

2. A disc herniated into the foramen of the nerve root may affect either the upper or the lower nerve roots.   **TRUE or FALSE**

3. A disc that is herniated far laterally will affect the lower nerve roots.

     TRUE or FALSE

4. Indications for discectomy include:

     1. Radicular pain

     2. Prominent radicular signs with modest axial pain

     3. Axial pain only

     4. Failure of conservative measures for at least 3 months

     5. Foot drop with bowel and bladder dysfunction

     6. Instability (Spondylolisthesis)

     7. 1,2, and 3

     8. All of the above

     9. Some of the above (circle the right answers)

Extremity Pain

1. Please complete the following:

    a. Nociceptive pain is characterized by

    b. Neuropathic pain is characterized by

    c. Central pain is characterized by

2. List at least three causes of shoulder impingement in an adult.

      i.

      ii.

      iii.

    b. Describe Yergason's test? What does it indicate?

3. Please match the referral pattern to its associated organ:

Organ	Referred Location
1. Appendix	____ Right shoulder
2. Bladder	____ Left chest, neck, arm, mouth, and spine from T4-7
3. Uterus	____ Spine below kidney, right lateral thigh, right chest at lower sternum
4. Ovaries	____ Same as heart but to the right side of body
5. Kidneys	____ Lateral skin over ovaries
6. Gallbladder	____ Anterior band across the pelvis, groin, and genitals
7. Liver	____ Neck from C3-6
8. Stomach	____ Sacrum from S2 to upper medial thigh
9. Lung & diaphragm	____ Right hypogastric area
10. Heart	____ Midline epigastric area and spine from T7-9

4. Trochanteric bursitis can be diagnosed using the maneuver shown below. What is the name of this test?

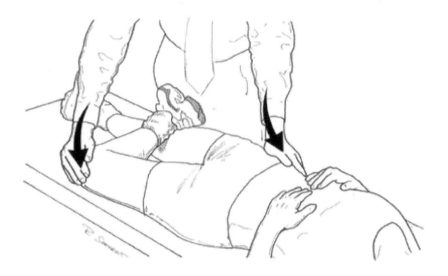

a. Name at least three treatment options for Trochanteric bursitis. How much weight is alleviated when a walker is utilized as compared to a cane?

Facial Pain

1. Trigeminal Neuralgia (TN):

   a. Determine if the statements below are true or false:

      i. TN is defined by paroxysmal attacks affecting one or more divisions of the trigeminal nerve. **TRUE or FALSE**

      ii. The attacks last from minutes to hours. **TRUE or FALSE**

      iii. Usually a clinically evident neurological deficit can be identified. **TRUE or FALSE**

      iv. The pain can be precipitated from trigger areas or by trigger factors. **TRUE or FALSE**

      v. TN can be attributed to another disorder and the headache lasts less than three months after successful treatment of the causative disorder. **TRUE or FALSE**

      vi. Often there is a sensory deficit on testing. **TRUE or FALSE**

vii. The V_2 branch is most commonly involved. **TRUE or FALSE**

b. Fill in the blanks for the statements below regarding TN:

   i. This is a disease of older individuals (>60 years old) except those patients with _____.

   ii. It is most commonly caused by compression of _____, but it can also be due to a demyelinating disease such as _____.

   iii. The disease is most responsive to _____.

   iv. Surgical treatment of choice is _____.

2. Atypical Trigeminal Neuralgia:

   a. How is Atypical TN different from Trigeminal Neuralgia?

3. Trigeminal Neuropathic pain:

   a. What physical examination finding sets Trigeminal Neuropathic pain apart from the other trigeminal disorders?

4. Other pain syndromes:

   a. Raeder's syndrome is associated with:

      1. Cluster headaches

      2. Constant pain and lesions such as aneurysms, tumors, trauma, infections, carotid artery dissections.

      3. Pathology of the first branch of the trigeminal nerve.

      4. Ptosis, miosis and an aching pain in the eye.

      5. 1, 2, and 3 are true

      6. 2 and 4 are true

      7. All are true

   b. Temporomandibular Joint pain is:

      1. Exacerbated with chewing.

      2. Evident by a palpable clicking when the TMJ is palpated through the external ear canal.

      3. Treated with splints, physical therapy, & acupuncture.

      4. Treated with Opioids, and cognitive or behavioral therapy (CBT).

      5. 1, 2, and 3 are correct

      6. 2 and 4 is correct

      7. All are correct

   c. Glossopharyngeal Neuralgia is characterized by:

      1. Treatment is similar to Trigeminal Neuralgia.

      2. The vagus nerve is always involved leading to bradycardia, or transient asystole.

(see next page for more answers)

3. Severe pain in the region of the tonsillar fossa.

4. It is not caused by demyelinating disorders.

5. 1 and 3 are true

6. All are true

d. Geniculate (Otalgic) Neuralgia is characterized by:

1. Severe pain deep in the tympanic membrane

2. It may be caused by herpes zoster and involve the facial nerve.

3. Patients may present with Ramsey-Hunt Syndrome.

4. 1 and 2 are true

5. All are true

6. I have no idea what Ramsey-Hunt Syndrome is!

e. Temporal Arteritis is:

1. Characterized by pain lasting from days to weeks.

2. Associated with Polymyalgia Rheumatica and an elevated ESR

3. Treatment includes steroid injection around the artery.

4. Is associated with jaw claudication, fever, malaise, anorexia, weight loss.

5. May lead to visual decline if untreated.

6. 1 and 3 are correct

7. 2 and 4 are correct

8. All are correct

Functional Impairment, Disability, & Handicap

1. Impairment is defined by the WHO as any _____ or abnormality of psychological, physical, or anatomic _____.

   a. The AMA Guides defines this as a condition which interferes with performance in activities of daily living.　　　**TRUE or FALSE**

   b. The AMA Guides provides subjective methods to evaluate and rate abnormalities.　　　**TRUE or FALSE**

   c. AMA Guides rate the level of impairment & then convert the value to a percentage relative to the body as a whole.　　　**TRUE or FALSE**

   d. The Diagnostic Related Estimates (DRE) helps to objectify the level of impairment to the body as a whole.　　　**TRUE or FALSE**

2. Disability is defined by the AMA Guides and the WHO as the _____ of a person's _____to perform due to an impairment.

a. Legal Disability is defined as the inability to meet social or occupational demands. **TRUE or FALSE**

b. Medicare Disability is determined by an administrative law judge. **TRUE or FALSE**

c. Social Security Administration defines disability as the inability to engage in ANY substantial work activity. **TRUE or FALSE**

d. AMA Guides define handicap as a condition where compensation must be used to overcome an impairment. **TRUE or FALSE**

e. What is the Katz Index?

3. Briefly describe the functionality measurement tools listed below:
    a. SF 36:

    b. Oswestry Disability Index:

    c. Pain Disability Index:

    d. The Functional Status Questionnaire (FSQ):

    e. The Functional Independence Measure (FIM):

Geriatric Pain

1. Physiologic changes:

   a. The elderly experience an increased tolerance of electrical current, cold, and mechanical pressure. **TRUE or FALSE**

   b. Acetylcholine is synthesized in interneurons and long projection neurons found in the nucleus basalis of Meynert, and the pedunculo-pontine nucleus. **TRUE or FALSE**

   c. Cholinergic projections reach the cerebral cortex, the limbic system, the Hippocampus, and the basal ganglia. **TRUE or FALSE**

   d. List at least two forms of therapy for Alzheimer's disease.

   e. The liver's regenerative capacity, microsomal hydroxylation, oxidation, glucuronidation, and non-microsomal oxidation are all decreased in the elderly. **TRUE or FALSE**

f. Renal vascular changes result in decreased renal blood flow, and reduced GFR. **TRUE or FALSE**

g. The volume of distribution decreases due to a decrease in lean body mass. **TRUE or FALSE**

2. Diagnosis, therapy, and pharmacology:

a. The Short Form McGill Questionnaire is used to assess the level of _____ in individuals.

b. A Functional Pain Scale can be used when _____ is more difficult.

c. The Katz Index is a tool used to assess the ability to perform ADLs and is most effective in _____ and the _____.

d. Pharmacologic treatment in the elderly:

i. Both selective and nonselective COX inhibitors have renal effects. **TRUE or FALSE**

ii. Aspirin is safer from a cardiovascular standpoint due to its affects on prostaglandins and thromboxane. **TRUE or FALSE**

iii. NSAIDs can lead to fluid retention and CHF by inhibiting Prostaglandin function. **TRUE or FALSE**

iv. NSAIDs pose an increased risk of renal damage especially in low flow states, GI bleed, and CHF. **TRUE or FALSE**

v. Celecoxib is: (circle the correct answers)
1. Indicated for OA, RA as well as acute pain in adults.
2. Eliminated predominantly by renal metabolism.
3. Has the ability to thwart prostacycline functionality in vascular endothelium while leaving thromboxane intact.
4. Decreases the risk of vasoconstriction, platelet aggregation, and thrombosis.

vi. Tricyclic Antidepressants increase the risk of orthostatic _____ and have anticholinergic effects.

vii. The safest TCA agent in the elderly is _____.

viii. Morphine metabolites include _____ and _____.

ix. Which of these morphine metabolites is more potent?

x. Oxycodone has a shorter T ½ in the younger patients compared to the elderly. **TRUE or FALSE**

xi. The controlled release formulation of Oxycodone has one active metabolite and should be used in a reduced dose in the elderly. **TRUE or FALSE**

xii. Dose reduction does not need to occur if Creatinine clearance is greater than 60 ml/min.   **TRUE or FALSE**

xiii. Meperidine is a poor choice for the elderly because it can cause cognitive effects due its _____,

xiv. Meperidine has an active metabolite called _____ which is hepatically excreted.   **TRUE or FALSE**

3. General health status:
   a. The leading cause of death in the elderly is:
      1. Heart disease
      2. Malignancies
      3. Cerebrovascular disease
      4. Pulmonary disease (COPD)

   b. Regarding Rheumatoid Arthritis in the elderly:
      1. The majority of patients have cervical spine involvement
      2. The lumbar spine is usually involved
      3. The cervical spine involvement includes Atlanto-Axial subluxation, vertical subluxation, and subaxial subluxation
      4. 1 and 3 are true
      5. All are true

c. Polymyalgia Rheumatica: (circle the correct statements)
   1. Affects patients older than 55 years of age, females, and Caucasians of northern European descent
   2. It is characterized by an inflammatory reaction that affects the proximal muscles
   3. Is associated with Temporal Arteritis
   4. The ESR is usually elevated (greater than 50)
   5. CK, EMG, and muscle biopsy are abnormal
   6. It responds well to low dose steroids

d. Temporal Arteritis (TA) is more common in females, and is associated with Polymyalgia Rheumatica.　　**TRUE or FALSE**

e. TA, if untreated, can lead to ischemic optic neuritis and blindness.
TRUE or FALSE

f. Post Herpetic Neuralgia is pain that persists 1-3 months after the rash from Herpes Zoster has healed.　PHN never really improves with time.
TRUE or FALSE

g. Dementia is characterized by:
   1. Generalized limitation of cognitive function.
   2. It is usually progressive
   3. If the consciousness is depressed, the patient is likely suffering from delirium.
   4. There is depression of consciousness.
   5. 1, 2, and 3 are correct
   6. All are true

h. Alzheimer's disease is characterized by:

    1. Acetylcholine-acetyltransferase depletion

    2. A slowly progressive degenerative process

    3. Neurofibrillary tangles and neuritic plaques

    4. There is a pathognomonic clinical presentation

    5. 1, 2, and 3 are true

    6. All are true

i. Parkinson's is associated with:

    1. Dopamine deficiency and cognitive deficit

    2. Pain due to dystonia and bradykinesia

    3. Disruption of cholinergic and dopaminergic tone at the basal ganglia

    4. Muscarinic antagonists are not useful in Parkinson's

    5. 1,2, and 3 are true

    6. All are true

Headaches

1. What is the difference between primary and secondary headaches?

2. Migraines:
    a. Migraine without aura is characterized by: (circle correct statements)
        i. At least 5 attacks, headaches lasting 4-72 hours and occurring <15 days a month.
        ii. Bilateral location with a pulsating quality
        iii. During the headache the patient experiences nausea or vomiting
        iv. During the headache the patient experiences photophobia or phonophobia.

    b. Migraine with aura is characterized by: (circle correct statement)
        i. At least 2 attacks fulfilling the symptoms for migraine
        ii. Irreversible visual or sensory, or speech symptoms
        iii. Motor weakness
        iv. Visual or sensory phenomena
        v. Development within 60 minutes of the aura
        vi. Symptom lasting more than 5 minutes and less than 60 minutes

c. Explain the neurovascular theory as it relates to the etiology of Migraines? (used the term trigeminal nucleus caudalis in your explanation)

d. The aura of Migraine is typically a _____ aura. The aura phase of migraines is thought to be associated with a reduction of cerebral blood flow in the gray matter of the posterior part of the hemisphere contralateral to the affected _____ field.

e. There are two approaches utilized for the treatment of Migraines. One is called _____ and the other is called _____.

f. Differentiate between the two modalities of Migraine treatment mentioned above. Utilize the term "Midas Disability Assessment Questionnaire" in your answer.

g. There are two general types of pharmacological treatments for migraines, abortive and prophylactic. Give examples of abortive drug categories?

h. Combining SSRI and SNRI with Triptans can result in a syndrome called _____.

i. Triptans inhibit the 5HT-1D receptors on nerve cells, and cause vasoconstriction by inhibiting the 5HT-1B receptors on blood vessels.

TRUE or FALSE

j. Prophylactic Migraine therapy includes beta blockers, calcium channel blockers, anticonvulsants, Botox, and Methysergide.

TRUE or FALSE

k. Simple analgesics with caffeine containing compounds and NSAIDS can be used for migraine treatment. **TRUE or FALSE**

3. Tension headaches:
   a. Tension type headaches: (circle correct statements)
      i. Can be episodic or chronic
      ii. Episodic tension headaches are defined as headaches occurring fewer than 15 days a month,
      iii. Chronic tension headaches occur 15 days or more a month for at least 6 months.
      iv. Tension headaches can last from minutes to weeks.
      v. There may be accompanying nausea or vomiting
      vi. Photophobia or phonophobia may occur
      vii. Unilateral location is typical, and is aggravated by physical activity
      viii. There is no prodrome or aura related to this headache type

b. Give examples of prophylactic and acute treatment for tension headaches. What are the criteria for prophylaxis treatment?

4. Trigeminal Autonomic Cephalgias:

   a. Cluster headaches are characterized by autonomic symptoms. What are these symptoms?

   b. Cluster headaches are classified as vascular headaches. The intense pain is caused by the dilation of blood vessels which creates pressure on _____. Among the most widely accepted theories is that cluster headaches are due to an abnormality in the _____ hence explaining the circadian pattern to the headaches.

   c. List at least two treatment options for acute Cluster headaches:

      1.

      2.

   d. List at least two prophylactic treatment options and two long term prophylactic treatment options for Cluster headaches.

      1.
      2.
      3.
      4.

e. A chronic cluster headache is sometimes referred to as _____ Continua.

f. SUNCT syndrome is identified as a unilateral headache occurring 5-30 times per hour primarily in the V_1 distribution and responsive to Carbamazepine. **TRUE or FALSE**

5. "Other" primary headaches:
   a. Primary Chronic Daily Headaches (CDH) are defined as headaches occurring greater than 15 days per month, related to structural or systemic disease. **TRUE or FALSE**

   b. New Daily Persistent Headache (NDPH) occurs greater than 15 days per month for more than one month and in a constant location. **TRUE or FALSE**

   c. In evaluating primary versus secondary headaches, what is the most important aspect of such an evaluation?

   d. Red flags in the evaluation of headaches include:
      1. Sudden onset. One should always perform an LP to further diagnose the etiology.
      2. Subacute headaches with increasing frequency or severity.

(see next page for more answers)

3. Headaches always presenting on the same side

4. Chronic daily headaches

5. 1, 2, and 3 are correct

6. 2, 3, and 4 are correct

7. All are correct

Neurolysis

1. Chemical Neurolysis:

    a. Phenol:

        i. What is the typical concentration of Phenol in aqueous mixture?

        ii. How does Phenol exert its effects? What is the baricity of Phenol?

        iii. Phenol has a shorter duration of action and produces a less intense blockade as compared to Alcohol.   **TRUE or FALSE**

    b. Alcohol:

        i. What is the typical concentration of Alcohol in solution?

        ii. Does Alcohol have the same mechanism of action as Phenol?

        iii. What is the baricity of Alcohol?

iv. Alcohol is the preferred neurolytic agent for

_____ malignancies.

v. If an Alcohol concentration greater than 50% is used in

neurolytic procedures, _____ and

_____can occur.

2. List at least two complication of neurolysis:

a.

b.

3. What is Anesthesia Dolorosa? Which neurolytic agent is more likely to produce this condition?

4. Subarachnoid Neurolysis:

a. If Alcohol is used, the patient is positioned in a

_____ position. If Phenol in Glycerin is used, the patient is positioned in a _____ position.

5. Superior Hypogastric Plexus:

a. The superior Hypogastric plexus is found anterior to the _____ vertebral bodies.

6. Ganglion Impar:
    a. This is a solitary terminal ganglion of the sympathetic chain. It is located anterior to the _____ and receives _____ input from rectal, bladder, and cervical regions. It is blocked when there is intractable pelvic pain.

7. Radiofrequency Lesioning:
    a. An individual facet is innervated by which medial branch nerves?

    b. In the lumbar region the medial branch block is performed at _____point.

    c. Why is the SI joint difficult to denervate?

    d. Cervical RF is achieved by placing the RF needle at the _____ of the trapezoid shaped articular process at the desired level and the level _____.

    e. Sensory and motor stimulation is performed to assess correct needle placement. Sensory stimulation is performed at _____Hz and motor stimulation is done at _____ Hz.

8. Cryoanalgesia:

    a. What are some indications for this technique?

    b. An "ice ball" is formed due to the _____ effect that is 0.5 cm for a 1.2 mm tip probe, and 1 cm for a 2 mm tip probe.

    c. Name at least three factors that determine the size of the ice ball formed at the tip of the cryoprobe.

    d. Briefly describe the Joule-Thomson effect.

    e. The advantage of the cryolesion over radiofrequency is that in this technique the _____ and the _____ remain intact.

Neuromuscular Syndromes

1. Myofascial Pain Syndrome (MPS):

   a. How is Myofascial Pain Syndrome different from Fibromyalgia?

   b. MPS is a chronic pain syndrome that affects a _____ part of the body.

   c. This syndrome is characterized by "tender points" on exam.

   TRUE or FALSE

   d. These hyper-irritable spots can give rise to a characteristic referred pain and tenderness over a wider area.   **TRUE or FALSE**

   e. Some of the major criteria for the diagnosis of MPS include:

      1. Weakness
      2. Autonomic dysfunction
      3. Referred pain, paresthesias or altered sensation
      4. 1 and 3 are true
      5. All are true

2. Fibromyalgia:

    a. Is a widespread painful condition involving 11/18 "trigger points" in specific areas. **TRUE or FALSE**

    b. There is an association with irritable bowel syndrome, SLE, RA, and Sjogren's syndrome. **TRUE or FALSE**

    c. This condition is often characterized by the presence of axial skeletal pain. **TRUE or FALSE**

    d. Name nine of the 18 painful sites needed for diagnosis of this condition.

    e. Digital palpation should be performed with an approximate force of _____ kg.

3. A Juvenile Primary Fibromyalgia syndrome also exists. Describe the criteria needed to diagnose this condition.

    a. Describe three adjuvant treatment options for this condition.

b. General concepts shared regarding the treatment of both MFP and Fibromyalgia include:

1. Improving motor dysfunction through physical therapy
2. Cardiovascular exercise
3. Restore normal sleep
4. 1 and 3 are correct
5. All are correct

4. Scapulo-costal Syndrome is a myofascial syndrome characterized by pain originating in the _____ of the scapula and radiating to the neck, back, arms, or chest wall.

5. What is the name of this maneuver and what does it test?

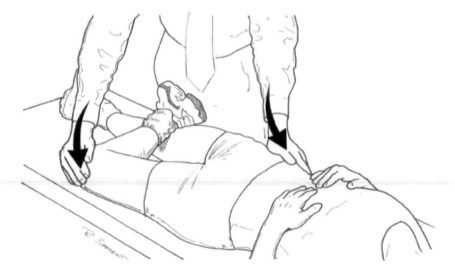

6.   What is the name of this maneuver and what does it test?

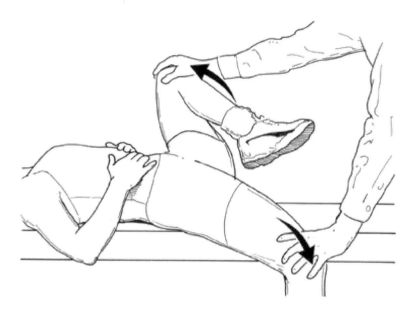

7.   What is the name of this maneuver and what does it test?

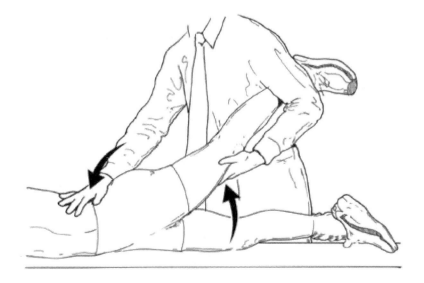

Neuropathic Pain

1. Mechanisms of Neuropathic pain:

   a. Describe deafferentation. How does it cause neuropathic pain?

      i. In a brachial plexus avulsion injury, the central processes remain _____ and there is increased activity in the dynamic range neurons in Rexed lamina _____.

      ii. How is the classic avulsion injury diagnosed?

      iii. The treatment of choice for a brachial plexus avulsion injury is the _____ procedure. What are some of the complications associated with this technique?

b. Describe loss of segmental inhibition. How does it cause neuropathic pain?

i. Loss of segmental inhibition is a purely peripheral lesion.

TRUE or FALSE

ii. Large fibers are more sensitive to decreased perfusion. Loss of these fibers eliminates the feedback mechanism and hence loss of inhibitory signals. **TRUE or FALSE**

iii. Segmental inhibition is how a TENS unit works.

TRUE or FALSE

iv. Give two examples of a nerve entrapment neuropathy.

v. What is Ramsey-Hunt syndrome?

vi. The Facial nerve stems from the _____ ganglion whereas the Trigeminal nerve stems from the _____ ganglion.

c. Describe ectopic impulse generation. How does it cause neuropathic pain?

    i. What is a Neuroma and how is it formed?

    ii. Schwann cells form a cord within which the axon grows at a rate of 10 mm/day. **TRUE or FALSE**

    iii. Neuromas are derived from primary afferent A-fibers. **TRUE or FALSE**

    iv. Focal demyelinating nerve injuries occur in primary afferent A-fibers. **TRUE or FALSE**

    v. The most common location of involvement in Trigeminal Neuralgia is V_2 and V_3. **TRUE or FALSE**

    vi. The etiology of Tic Douloureux is believed to be compression of the fifth cranial nerve by _____ as it leaves the pons in the subarachnoid space towards _____.

1. The treatment of choice for Trigeminal Neuralgia is

   _____.

2. Patients presenting with Trigeminal Neuralgia may be suffering from a focal demyelinating disease called

   _____.

2. Phantom limb pain:
   a. The mechanisms of phantom limb pain include:
      1. Deafferentation
      2. Ectopic impulse generation
      3. Ephapses
      4. Neuroplasticity
      5. 1 and 3 are correct
      6. 2 and 4 are correct
      7. All are correct

3. Define the following neuropathic terms:
   a. Hyperalgesia:
   b. Allodynia:
   c. Hyperpathia:
   d. Dysesthesia:
   e. Paresthesia:
   f. Hyperesthesia:

4. Poly-Neuropathy:

    a. Polyneuropathy involves nerve fibers of all sizes.

             TRUE or FALSE

    b. Polyneuropathy can result in both sensory and motor changes.

             TRUE or FALSE

    c. Axonotmesis result in a distal burning and pins and needles sensation.

             TRUE or FALSE

    d. Acute Inflammatory Demyelinating Polyneuropathy (AIDP) presents with proximal dysesthesias, while Chronic Inflammatory Demyelinating Polyneuropathy (CIDP) frequently presents more distal rather than proximal.   **TRUE or FALSE**

    e. Under what conditions are nerve biopsies indicated?

Neurophysiology

1. Electromyography determines the integrity of the _____ motor neuron from the anterior horn cell to the muscle. Both EMG and NCV are used to determine the integrity of the _____ nervous system.

    a. List at least three conditions in which an EMG exam may be helpful.

    b. The EMG exam helps distinguish between neuropathy, radiculopathy, myopathy, and motor neuron disease.   **TRUE or FALSE**

2. Peripheral neuropathies associated with pain include:
   1. Diabetes mellitus
   2. Guillain-Barre Syndrome
   3. Amyloidosis
   4. Fabry's disease
   5. 1 and 3 are correct
   6. 2 and 4 are correct
   7. All are correct

3. There are four components to the EMG exam, what are they?

        i.

        ii.

        iii.

        iv.

4. In myopathic conditions, an increased amount of insertional activity may be found and fiber recruitment may be out of proportion to effort.

TRUE or FALSE

5. EMG findings in neuropathic conditions immediately post nerve or neuropathic insult my show no abnormality.   **TRUE or FALSE**

6. If denervation has occurred, fibrillations will occur in as early as _____weeks.

7. Nerve Conduction Velocity testing (NCV) measures:

    a. A-delta fiber velocity

    b. A-beta fiber velocity

    c. C fiber velocity

    d. a and c are correct

    e. b is correct

8. NCV testing is useful in small fiber neuropathy.   **TRUE or FALSE**

9. Complete the missing information in the table below:

Fiber	Function	Diameter (micrometer)	Velocity (m/s)	Refractory Period (ms)
Aβ (myelinated)			30-70	0.4-1
Aδ (myelinated)			12-30	1.2
C (unmyelinated)			0.1-2.5	2-50

10. What is Current Perception Threshold (CPT) testing?

11. Quantitative Sudomotor Axon Reflex Test (QSART) is used to assess the _____ nerve fibers which are linked to sweat glands.

Neurosurgical Invasive Techniques

1. Surgical procedures:

    a. Why is peripheral nerve ablation increasingly uncommon?

    b. Peripheral nerve ablation is mainly used for _____
        neuralgia.

    c. The DREZ procedure is mainly used in _____, or
        in patients with spinal cord injury transitional zone pain.

    d. Cordotomy is used to relieve _____ extremity pain due to
        cancer.

    e. Commissural myelotomy is used for _____ cancer related pain.

    f. Punctate midline myelotomy is used to treat _____ and
        rectal related cancer pain.

2. Augmentative procedures:

   a. Intrathecal (IT) pumps deliver medicine directly into the CNS. This is the mainstay for _____ pain.

   b. The advantage of intrathecal drug delivery over epidural delivery is that the dose of the drug can be decreased by a factor of 10.

      TRUE or FALSE

   c. Morphine induced hyperalgesia can occur when IT morphine dose is greater than _____ mg/day.

   d. Complete the missing information in the table below which illustrates the maximum recommended IT dosage of some common drugs:

Drug	Dosage (mg/day)	Conc. (mg/ml)
Morphine		30
Hydromorphone		30
Bupivacaine		38
Clonidine		2.0

   e. Morphine and _____ are the only drugs that are FDA approved for use in pain pumps.

f. Prialt (Ziconotide) blocks the _____ found on neuronal cell bodies.

g. Electrical stimulation is a direct result of Melzack and Wall's gate control theory and is best utilized for _____ pain.

h. Electrical stimulation is also used for ischemic leg pain, and angina (both of which are not FDA approved). **TRUE or FALSE**

i. There is no evidence that spinal cord stimulation works well for nociceptive pain. **TRUE or FALSE**

j. Spinal cord stimulation modulates laminae I, II, and V as well as GABA, Glycine, 5-HT, and Substance P. **TRUE or FALSE**

Nociceptive Pain

1. Upper extremity and Neck Pain:

    a. Complete the missing information in the table below which lists the signs
    and symptoms of nerve root compression of the cervical region:

Location	Referred Pain	Motor Dysfxn	Sensory Dysfxn	Reflex changes
C5				
C6				
C7				
C8				N/A

b. Where does the vertebral artery travel in the cervical region? Why shouldn't one block the facet joint at the cervical level?

c. Acute localized pain due to an acute HNP resolves spontaneously in 75% of cases. **TRUE or FALSE**

2. Low Back Pain:

a. Most causes of LBP are due to ligamentous strain and not degenerative disks, or HNP. **TRUE or FALSE**

b. Majority of LBP originates from the PLL, facet joints, and deep muscles. Most LBP resolves within 2 months. **TRUE or FALSE**

c. Imaging studies only accurately assess facet joint, nerve root, or annular tear of discs. **TRUE or FALSE**

d. Describe at least three pathological findings that plain X-rays in PA and lateral views can show:

   1.

   2.

   3.

e. Describe at least one indication for Myelography.

f. Disks make up _____ of the height of the vertebral column in the lumbar region, and _____ of the height in the cervical and thoracic regions.

g. The PLL narrows at the levels _____ and is less able to limit a postero-lateral HNP.

h. The Majority of HNPs occur at which levels?

i. Disks are highly innervated in the exterior ____ by _____ nerves, dorsal ramus, and the sympathetic nerves. A disk rupture into the vertebral body is called a _____.

j. In the lumbar region the L3 nerve root exits at the _____ intervertebral foramen. This is different in the cervical region where the C6 nerve root exits at the _____ intervertebral foramen.

k. In the lumbar region, the nerve roots run caudally along the posterior vertebral body before exiting the intervertebral foramen. Hence, a HNP at L4-5 will "catch" the _____ nerve root.

l. Complete the missing information in the table below which illustrates the significance of the level of HNP and the physical exam findings:

HNP	Nerve Root involved	Pain	Numbness	Weakness	Atrophy	Reflexes
L3-4		LB, Hip, postero-lateral thigh, anterior leg	Anteromedial thigh and knee		Quadriceps	
L4-5		SIJ, Hip, lateral thigh & leg	Lateral leg, toes 1-3		Minor	
L5-S1		SIJ, hip, postero-lateral thigh, leg to heel	Back of calf, lateral heel, big toe		Gastrocnemius, soleus	

m. Facet Joint Disease (FJD) usually presents with:

1. Gluteal or thigh pain
2. The pain is typically unilateral in the lumbar region
3. There is radiation of pain to the back of the thigh or knee
4. Symptoms are aggravated by hyperextension or lateral flexion
5. 1 and 3 are correct
6. 2 and 4 are correct
7. All are correct

n. Disk injury increases Phospholipase A2 (PLA-2) liberation which in turn liberates Arachidonic acid from cell membranes. This process can be reversed by steroids and NSAIDs.   **TRUE or FALSE**

o. How is chronic pain defined?

p. Regarding discogenic LBP, 70% improve within _____ with conservative treatment and 90% improve in _____.

q. Spinal stimulation techniques involve modifying small pain fiber input (C and A-delta) by faster A-alpha or A-beta neural input.

                    TRUE or FALSE

3. Musculoskeletal Pain:

a. Myofascial pain is synonymous with:

    1. Myositis
    2. Fibromyalgia pain
    3. Fibrositis
    4. Myofascitis
    5. 1 and 3 are correct
    6. 2 and 4 are correct
    7. All are correct

b. What is the difference between muscle mechano-receptors and chemo-receptors?

c. Trigger points are a hallmark of what type of condition?

d. Which of the following statements accurately describes the pathology of a trigger point:

    1. There is rupture of the SR and release of calcium

    2. Depletion of ATP leads to electrical silence

    3. Local ischemia, hypoxia, and release of algogenic substances occurs

    4. Nociceptive sensitization and CNS stimulation results in increased sympathetic activity, and local tissue ischemia

    5. 1 and 3 are correct

    6. 2 and 4 are correct

    7. All are correct

e. The process that involves transfer of ionized substances through intact skin is called _____.

f. Most skeletal pain is noted in the joints which are richly endowed with nerve fibers. Immunologic disorders are typically mono-articular while inflammatory disorders are poly-articular.   **TRUE or FALSE**

g. Tender points are the hallmark of which disease condition?

h. The tender points are palpated bilaterally with _____ kg of pressure and are typically at the muscle-tendon junctions.   **TRUE or FALSE**

Obstetrical Pain

1. Innervation of pelvic organs:

   a. The lower pelvic structures have a dual innervation which includes:

      1. Afferent sympathetics

      2. Efferent sympathetics

      3. Parasympathetics

      4. 1 and 3 are true

      5. All are true

   b. The autonomic innervation of the pelvis is conducted by the:

      1. Superior Hypogastric plexus

      2. Inferior Hypogastric plexus

      3. Ganglion Impar

      4. 1 and 3 are true

      5. All are true

   c. The Hypogastric nerve connects which two structures?

   d. The Superior Hypogastric plexus is mostly parasympathetic.

   TRUE or FALSE

e. The Inferior Hypogastric plexus contains sympathetic fibers which originate from the pelvic splanchnics. **TRUE or FALSE**

f. Pelvic splanchnics are parasympathetic fibers derived from the ventral rami of spinal nerves S2-S4. **TRUE or FALSE**

g. The Ganglion Impar is the distal extension of the sacral sympathetic chain. **TRUE or FALSE**

h. The uterine body and fundus are innervated by the superior and inferior hypogastric plexuses. **TRUE or FALSE**

i. The cervix is innervated by the inferior hypogastric plexus (derived from S2-S4). **TRUE or FALSE**

j. Afferent nerves from the uterine-cervical area travel through the inferior hypogastric plexus to the T10-L2 spinal segments.

TRUE or FALSE

k. The A-delta and C afferent nerve fibers accompany the parasympathetic nerves from the uterine and cervical plexus to the superior hypogastric plexus. **TRUE or FALSE**

l. The upper ¾ of the vagina is innervated by the uterovaginal plexus and the sacral fibers S2-S4, and the lower ¼ is innervated by the sacral nerve that travels via the pudendal nerve. **TRUE or FALSE**

m. The bladder, rectum, anus, and perineum have a dual innervation.

TRUE or FALSE

2. Pain pathways in obstetric pain:

    a. Nociceptive stimuli during the first stage of labor are carried via afferent fibers through the _____ and _____ nerves.

    b. The second stage of labor is characterized by full cervical dilation to delivery. Nociception at this stage is carried out by the _____ nerves, _____ nerves (sacral S2-S4), and the _____ nerve.

    c. The third stage of labor is characterized by delivery of the placenta. Uterine contraction after delivery will carry nociception via _____ nerves.

3. Non-obstetric pain and pregnancy:

    a. Lumbar lordosis as well as ligament laxity 2nd to secretion of _____ in as early as 10-12 weeks gestation can lead to back pain.

    b. Secretion of _____ can also lead to increased SI joint mobility. The SI joint can refer pain to the _____ and _____ specifically during weight bearing.

    c. Although CT scanning should be avoided, MRI scans are felt to be safe in parturient patients.   **TRUE or FALSE**

4. Medications during pregnancy:

    a. These two large polar molecules do not cross the placenta to reach the fetus, they are _____ and _____.

    b. Name the four factors that determine whether a medication can transfer through the placenta to the fetus.

        i.

        ii.

        iii.

        iv.

    c. Organogenesis occurs between _____ to _____ weeks and this is most critical for minimizing medication exposure.

    d. Match the FDA classification to its relative teratogenecity:

Category A	_____ Contraindicated in pregnancy
Category B	_____ Risk cannot be ruled out
Category C	_____ Positive evidence of risk in humans
Category D	_____ Human studies show no fetal risk in any trimester
Category X	_____ Human studies show no evidence of risk

    e. Aspirin and NSAIDs:

        i. Prostaglandins trigger labor.   **TRUE or FALSE**

        ii. Aspirin and NSAIDs can prolong gestation and labor.

                TRUE or FALSE

iii. Aspirin use during pregnancy can lead to an increased risk of intracranial hemorrhage, & closure of ductus arteriosus.

TRUE or FALSE

iv. In the fetus, Indomethacin has been associated with neonatal renal failure, persistent pulmonary hypertension, necrotizing enterocolitis, and neonatal death. **TRUE or FALSE**

f. Anticonvulsants:

i. Phenytoin, Carbamazepine, or Valproic acid carry no increased risk of congenital defects in their fetus.

TRUE or FALSE

ii. What is Fetal Hydantoin Syndrome? Which medication can cause this condition and how does it do so?

iii. Depakote is associated with _____ when used in the first trimester.

iv. Valproic acid crosses the placenta and is excreted into human breast milk. **TRUE or FALSE**

g. Antidepressants:

    i. If the fetus is exposed to an SSRI in the third trimester, there is a risk for development of _____ in the newborn.

h. Benzodiazepines:

    i. Exposure in the first trimester can cause _____ & _____, and congenital hernias.

i. Steroids:

    i. While most corticosteroids cross the placenta, Prednisone and Prednisolone are _____ by the placenta.

j. Local anesthetics:

    i. Mexiletine is not lipid soluble and can not cross the placenta.

        TRUE or FALSE

k. Migraine medication:

    i. Ergotamines have significant teratogenic effects and can cause uterine contractions. **TRUE or FALSE**

    ii. Caffeine is associated with low birth weight babies.

        TRUE or FALSE

    iii. Beta blockers can cause low birth weight babies.

        TRUE or FALSE

5. Premature induction of labor:

    a. Acupuncture may produce version during breech presentation.

        TRUE or FALSE

6. Lactation and Medication:

   a. What is the neonatal exposure to the medication that crosses the placenta?

   b. When is breast milk synthesized? When should a lactating mother take her medication?

   c. Serotonin inhibits Dopamine which leads to increased Prolactin levels and increased lactation.   **TRUE or FALSE**

   d. Match the risk classification of maternal medication use during lactation with its definition:

      1. Category 1   _____ Compatible with breast feeding

      2. Category 2   _____ Should not be consumed during lactation

      3. Category 3   _____ Effects on newborn is unknown

   e. Medication use during lactation:
      i. Although NSAID transfer is limited by slow neonatal elimination, this category is considered safe.

                                        TRUE or FALSE

      ii. Acetaminophen does not enter breast milk, and has no teratogenic effects.   **TRUE or FALSE**

iii. Anticonvulsants such as Gabapentin have high breast milk concentrations. **TRUE or FALSE**

iv. Highly protein bound agents that have low breast milk concentrations include Phenytoin, Tiagabine (Gabitril), and Valproate (Depakote). **TRUE or FALSE**

v. Fluoxetine and Sertraline are preferred Antidepressant agents.

TRUE or FALSE

vi. TCAs should be avoided. **TRUE or FALSE**

vii. Benzodiazepines are safe agents despite the fact that their metabolites can be detected in breast milk.

TRUE or FALSE

viii. Opioids are all excreted into breast milk.

TRUE or FALSE

ix. Meperidine has an active metabolite called _____ which tends to accumulate in the neonate.

x. Ergotamines are associated with neonatal _____ and severe GI disturbances.

xi. Intra-operative Methergine for uterine atony is contraindicated for breast feeding. **TRUE or FALSE**

7. Diagnostic imaging during pregnancy:

    a. Pregnancy is an absolute contraindication to radiographic evaluation.

          TRUE or FALSE

    b. Is MRI safe during pregnancy?

    c. What is the best time to perform a radiographic exam if the patient is pregnant?

    d. During pregnancy contrast agents can be used in radiographic examinations.

          TRUE or FALSE

    e. Increased risk of malformations occurs above 10 rads of exposure (100 mGy, or 100 rem).   **TRUE or FALSE**

    f. If an embryo or fetus is exposed to radiation secondary to a diagnostic procedure, a therapeutic abortion should be considered.

          TRUE or FALSE

Painful Medical Conditions

1. AIDS:

   a. Pain syndromes related to AIDS include:

      1. Kaposi's sarcoma

      2. Reiter's syndrome

      3. Vasculitis

      4. 1 and 3 are correct

      5. All are correct

   b. HIV neuropathy is most commonly seen in what regions of the body?

   c. What is Kaposi's sarcoma?

2. Multiple Sclerosis (MS):

    a. MS is characterized by:

        1. An inflammatory destruction of CNS myelin

        2. An auto immune mediated destruction of axons

        3. The classic plaque lesion can appear anywhere

        4. The disease course is slowly progressive

        5. 1 and 3 are correct

        6. 2 and 4 are correct

    b. Diagnostic work up for MS includes:

        1. MRI of brain and spinal cord

        2. Identification of plaques that are > 3 mm

        3. CSF testing for IgG & myelin basic protein

        4. Detection of mononuclear pleocytosis

        5. 1 and 3 are correct

        6. All are correct

    c. Clinically patients suffer from:

        1. Mobility dysfunction (weakness, paresis, and spasticity)

        2. Incoordination (ataxia)

        3. Optic neuritis

        4. Bladder dysfunction

        5. Some of the above are true (circle correct answers)

        6. All of the above are true

    d. What is Lhermitte's sign? How does it relate to MS?

3. Amyotrophic Lateral Sclerosis (ALS):

    a. ALS is characterized as a progressive degeneration of

        _____. It is also called _____disease.

    b. Patients present with UMN and LMN signs.

                                  TRUE or FALSE

    c. Describe both upper motor neuron and lower motor neuron signs.

        i. UMN:

        ii. LMN:

4. Parkinson's Disease:

    a. This disease involves the loss of cells in:

        1. The Substantia Nigra

        2. The Locus Coeruleus

        3. The Putamen

        4. Only one of the above is correct (circle the answer)

        5. All of the above are true

    b. Pain and sensory symptoms precede the motor symptoms.

                                  TRUE or FALSE

5. Guillain-Barre Syndrome:

    a. This syndrome is characterized by:

        1. An immune inflammatory polyneuropathy

        2. Descending motor weakness

        3. It is triggered by CMV, EBV, or vaccinations

        4. Results in respiratory failure in 90% of cases

        5. 1 and 3 are correct

        6. 2 and 4 are correct

        7. All are correct

    b. Pain can precede the motor symptoms in this disease.

                                        TRUE or FALSE

6. Peripheral Vascular Disease (PVD):

    a. In the case of Thromboangiitis Obliterans (Buerger's disease) bilateral claudication can occur in the instep of feet or in the hands.

                                        TRUE or FALSE

7. Sickle Cell disease:

    a. What factors can exacerbate sickle cell disease? How is it treated?

8. Raynaud's disease:

    a. How is Raynaud's disease different from Reynaud's phenomenon?

b. Raynaud's disease presents bilaterally whereas Raynaud's phenomenon may be unilateral in presentation.

TRUE or FALSE

9. Systemic Lupus Erythematosus (SLE):

a. SLE can be characterized by:

1. Occurring secondary to Tegretol, or Dilantin use
2. Migratory polyarthritis of hands, wrists, and knees
3. Serositis of any serous containing cavity
4. Presentation of Nephritis, seizures and strokes
5. 1 and 3 are correct
6. All are correct

10. Osteoarthritis (OA) and Rheumatoid Arthritis (RA):

a. Differentiate between OA and RA.

b. RA occurs asymmetrically in weight bearing joints. Bony hypertrophy is often noted. **TRUE or FALSE**

c. In the case of OA, joint use leads to pain and inactivity leads to stiffness and pain relief. **TRUE or FALSE**

d. What are Heberden's nodes, and Bouchard's nodes?

e. RA occurs late in life, presents with symmetrical pain in small joints with bony erosions on x-ray. **TRUE or FALSE**

f. Felty's syndrome is characterized by 3 conditions. What are they?

    i.

    ii.

    iii.

11. Seronegative Spondylo-Arthropathies:

a. How are the seronegative spondylo-arthropathies different from RA?

b. What is Ankylosing spondylitis? Name two extra-articular manifestations of this condition.

c. Reiter's syndrome is:

    1. An autoimmune condition that develops in response to an infection in another part of the body

    2. Characterized by urethritis, conjunctivitis, uveitis, asymmetric arthritis, & sacroiliitis.

    3. Associated with HLA-B27

    4. Some of the above are true (circle correct answers)

    5. None of the above are true

d. Patients with Polymyalgia Rheumatica (PMR) may complain of stiffness that is worse in the morning or after rest.

TRUE or FALSE

e. A 15% association with Temporal Arteritis exists in patients that are diagnosed with PMR.   **TRUE or FALSE**

12. Cardiac Pain:

   a. Prinzmetal's angina and Microvascular angina are similar in that they are both associated with _____ coronary arteries.

   b. Treatment with _____ is now the classic drug to be used with Syndrome X.

   c. It is normal to observe EKG changes such as ST elevation and upright T-waves in Acute Pericarditis.   **TRUE or FALSE**

   d. The incidence of aortic dissection is higher in males with Ehler Danlos syndrome.   **TRUE or FALSE**

13. Pulmonary Pain:

   a. Pulmonary embolism can occur due to hypercoagulable states such as: (circle correct answers)

      1. Protein C, and protein S deficiency
      2. Polycythemia
      3. Malignancy
      4. Obesity
      5. AT III deficiency

   b. What is the classic triad of symptoms associated with PE?

c. Please differentiate between an exudate and a transudate?

14. Gastrointestinal Pain:

    a. Esophageal dysmotility can cause substernal pain and radiating pain that mimics MI. Treatment for this condition includes:

        1. Nitroglycerin

        2. Calcium channel blockers

        3. Botulinum toxin

        4. Antidepressants

        5. 1 and 3 are correct

        6. 2 and 4 are correct

        7. All are correct

    b. There is a clear correlation between severity of symptoms and the extent of lesions in NSAID gastritis. **TRUE or FALSE**

    c. H. Pylori gastritis is treated with triple antibiotic therapy of (CAM) _____ and _____ and _____.

    d. Zollinger-Ellison syndrome is characterized by a _____ secreting tumor associated with non-β islet cell cancer of the _____.

15. Liver:

    a. Nociception in the liver is vagally mediated and vagotomy will relieve hepatic pain. **TRUE or FALSE**

    b. Fitz-Hugh Curtis syndrome is a venereal disease associated with _____ or _____ infections.

    c. Chronic pancreatitis evolves from either recurrent acute pancreatitis or "idiopathic" pancreatitis. **TRUE or FALSE**

    d. How is chronic pancreatitis best diagnosed?

16. Kidneys and Ureters:

    a. The kidneys are innervated by the sympathetic celiac and aortico-renal ganglion, the vagus, and visceral afferents (T10-T12).

                                                    TRUE or FALSE

    b. The upper 2/3 of the ureters receive the same innervation as the kidneys. **TRUE or FALSE**

    c. The lower 1/3 of the ureters receive innervation from the superior and inferior hypogastric plexuses and S2-S4. **TRUE or FALSE**

    d. Nephrolithiasis most commonly occurs due to _____ and _____ stones.

Pediatric Pain

1. CNS and Developmental Anatomy:

    a. Thalamocortical synapses occur by the 20-24th week of gestation. Spinothalamic myelination is complete by the _____ week of gestation.

    b. Neonates have a well developed nociceptive afferent system but the descending control pathways are developmentally delayed.

    TRUE or FALSE

    c. Which two receptors mediate fast excitatory transmission and are found in the newborn?

    d. This receptor is involved in slower post-synaptic processing and in persistent chronic pain states. It has widespread expression in the neonatal period. This is the _____ receptor.

    e. Glycine can bind to and provide tonic suppression of this receptor; this is the _____ receptor.

f. The two main inhibitory neurotransmitters in the nervous system are
_____ and _____.

2. Developmental abnormalities:

a. Spina Bifida Occulta is a defect of the vertebral arch and it is a neural tube defect most common at L5-S1.   **TRUE or FALSE**

b. Chiari Malformation is a neural tube defect that is characterized by the brain, and brainstem herniating through foramen Rotundum.

TRUE or FALSE

c. Arnold-Chiari Malformation is characterized by Spina Bifida and Meningomyelocele. Alpha-fetoprotein is a marker for this condition.

TRUE or FALSE

3. Pain Measurement:

a. Match the patient's age to the ability of expressing pain below:

a. 0-3 months   ____ May use the word "hurt", non cognitive coping strategies

b. 3-6 months   ____ Begins to describe pain and attributes external causes to it

c. 6-18 months   ____ Develops fear of painful situations, localization of pain is evident, will use words associated with pain

d. 18-24 months   ____ Can differentiate levels of pain & begin to use PCA pumps

e. 24-36 months   ____ Can explain why pain hurts

f. 36-60 months   ____ No apparent understanding of pain

g. 5-7 years   ____ Pain response is accompanied by sadness and anger

h. 7-10 years   ____ Gives gross indication of pain intensity, uses descriptive terms

i. 11 years   ____ Can explain the value of pain

b. Complete the blanks for each of the statements below:

    i. Behavioral observation is used in _____ and children under _____ years of age.

    ii. McGrath scale is useful in children that are _____ years old.

    iii. Analogue chromatic scales are used in children age _____ years.

    iv. Faces scales is useful in children _____ years old.

    v. Numeric Rating Scales (NRS) and Visual Analogue Scales (VAS) can be used in children that are _____ years and older.

    vi. The Oucher scale is used for children of ages _____ and involves the use of numbers as well as actual children faces.

    vii. The CHEOPS scale utilizes behavioral assessment in _____ and _____ to assess pain.

    viii. The CHEOPS scale is a useful tool for assessing post operative pain levels in pediatric patients. **TRUE or FALSE**

    ix. The DC Children's Hospital Pain and Discomfort scale is most appropriate for pediatric _____ use in children _____ years old.

4. Pediatric Pain Syndromes:

    a. In descending order, what are the three most common pain syndromes in children?

    b. Pediatric migraines may be accompanied by abdominal pain.

                                                       TRUE or FALSE

    c. Pediatric headaches are characterized by recurrent persistent early morning headaches.   **TRUE or FALSE**

    d. Pediatric migraines are typically unilateral in nature, accompanied by recurrent abdominal pain, and visual, sensory, or motor aura.

                                                       TRUE or FALSE

    e. Complicated migraines such as Hemiplegic migraines are those that present with neurologic signs and are considered normal in this age range.   **TRUE or FALSE**

    f. Circle the statement(s) which correctly indicate neuroimaging for further diagnosis of headaches in children:

        1. Focal neurologic signs during aura with fixed unilaterality
        2. Focal neurologic symptoms with headache
        3. Headache awakens patient from sleep
        4. Early morning headaches
        5. Migraine with seizure
        6. Child < 6 yrs old whose primary complaint is headache

g. What is the most common treatment regimen for pediatric patients with recurrent abdominal pain?

h. What is Osgood-Schlatter disease?

i. Juvenile Rheumatoid Arthritis is characterized by: (circle the correct answers)

1. The age of onset of less than 16 years old
2. Chronic synovitis
3. Articular erosions
4. Extra-articular manifestations

j. Back pain occurs in children almost as often as it does in adults. Except that it is often a sign of significant underlying disorder in children. **TRUE or FALSE**

k. What is Scheuermann's disease?

l. Pars interarticularis defect (spondylolysis) occurs with greatest incidence at which spinal level?

m. Give two examples of how Complex Regional Pain Syndrome is different in children as compared to adults.

5. Therapy:

    a. Which of the following statements regarding gastric physiology are correct?

        i. Gastric absorption of drugs in children is comparable to adults by 6 months of age.

        ii. Gastric emptying is delayed in infants less than 6 months of age.

        iii. Gastric acid production reaches adult levels by 3 years of age.

        iv. Protein binding is lower in the newborn due to lower albumin and α-1 glycoprotein levels.

        v. Local anesthetics are less protein bound in the newborn and the free fraction is increased, increasing the risk of fetal toxicity.

    b. How are ester local anesthetics metabolized?

    c. Do Neonates and infants have the same amount of adult plasma cholinesterase?

    d. Examples of ester local anesthetics include: (circle correct answers)

        1. Chlorprocaine

        2. Marcaine

        3. Procaine

        4. Cocaine

        5. Tetracaine

    e. In toddlers and children the analgesic clearance is delayed due to immature hepatic enzymes and decreased renal blood flow.

                         TRUE or FALSE

f. Premature infants and neonates have an increased level of blood brain barrier compared to adults.   **TRUE or FALSE**

g. Complete the missing information in the table below regarding analgesic doses in children:

Drug	Dose (mg/kg)	Infusion (mg/kg/hr)	Comment
Meperidine		Not recommended	*Avoid* with Renal insufficiency
Morphine		0.01	First choice
Hydromorphone		0.003	*Good* with Renal insufficiency
Fentanyl		0.0005	Short acting

h. Complete the missing information regarding PCA doses in children indicated in the table below:

Drug	Dose (mcg/kg)	Infusion (mcg/kg/hr)	4 hour limit (mcg/kg)
Morphine		5-10 (0.01 mg/kg/hr)	300 (0.3 mg/kg)
Hydromorphone		1-3 (0.003 mg/kg/hr)	60
Fentanyl		0.1 (0.0001 mg/kg/hr)	4

i. Review the pediatric starting doses of Acetaminophen, Ketorolac, and Nortriptyline before moving on to the next chapter!

Chapter 23

Pelvic Pain

1. Pelvic anatomy:

   a. There are two types of cartilage at the level of the SI joint. At the articular surface there is _____ cartilage and at the level of the Ilium there is _____ cartilage.

   b. The Superior Hypogastric Plexus (SHP) is formed by the union of which two structures?

   c. The SHP is located at the left ventral lateral border of _____. It has _____fibers that give branches to the ovarian and testicular plexuses.

   d. The Middle Hypogastric Plexus (MHP) is derived from the _____ hypogastric plexus. It acts as a bridge between the _____ and the _____.

   e. The MHP is joined by the lowest lumbar splanchnic nerves and sends branches to the ovarian/testicular plexuses, and the ureteral plexus.

   TRUE or FALSE

f. The Inferior Hypogastric Plexus (IHP) contains _____ efferents, afferents, and postganglionic sympathetic sacral splanchnic fibers.

g. The preganglionic sympathetic fibers originate from _____.

h. It also contains _____fibers from the pelvic splanchnic nerves, particularly the cell bodies of _____ of the spinal cord which synapse with the cell bodies of postganglionic neurons or walls of the viscera.

i. What is the Ganglion of Walther?

j. The Lumbar Plexus originates from _____ and gives rise to a number of nerves: (match the nerve to its nerve root source)

1.	Ilio-hypogastric n.	_____	L2-L4
2.	Ilio-inguinal n.	_____	L2-L4
3.	Genitofemoral n.	_____	L3-L4
4.	Lateral femoral cutaneous n.	_____	T12-L1
5.	Femoral n.	_____	L1-L2
6.	Obturator n.	_____	T12-L1

k. The Sacral plexus consists of two nerves. What are these two nerves?
   i.
   ii.

l. The Sciatic nerve arises from _____ and passes through the belly of the piriformis muscle as it travels toward the greater sciatic foramen.

m. The Pudendal nerve leaves the pelvis through the greater sciatic foramen and re-enters the pelvis through the lesser sciatic foramen and proceeds anteriorly through _____ canal which is derived from the Obturator internus muscle.

n. The Pudendal nerve arises from three branches which include the anterior primary rami of _____, _____, and all of _____.

2. In your own words, briefly describe Viscerosomatic or Visceromotor convergence.

3. Pelvic pain etiologies:

Provide a diagnosis based on the supplied descriptions. Several possible diagnosis options are offered below.

(Corpus luteum cyst, Twisted ovarian cyst, Cyclic pelvic pain, Primary dysmenorrhea, Secondary dysmenorrhea, Endometriosis, Adenomyosis, Pelvic Congestion, Ovarian remnant syndrome, Salpingo-oophoritis, Vaginismus, Tension myalgia, Bartholinitis, Skene's urethritis, Urethral syndrome, Interstitial cystitis, Osteitis pubis, Myofascial pain)

a. Local vascular blood supply is inhibited leading to sharp pain with radiation to the iliac fossa as well as N/V. _____

b. Associated with menstruation, primary or secondary dysmenorrhea. Up to 50% of females suffer from this disorder. _____

c. This is menstrual pain without pelvic pathology. Pain is suprapubic, referred to both thighs and lumbo-sacral spine. It can be accompanied by N/V, and diarrhea. Its onset is day 1 of menses and persists for 48-72 hours. _____

d. This is menstrual pain that is due to pelvic pathology. Examples of which include endometriosis, and adenomyosis. _____

e. After primary dysmenorrhea this is the second most common cause of chronic pelvic pain. It is defined by the presence of endometrial glands or stroma outside the uterus. _____

f. This is characterized by endometrial glands which embed themselves within the hyperplastic uterine muscle leading to heavy menses, dysmenorrhea, and an enlarged tender uterus. _____

g. Congestion of the arteries and the veins of the ovaries and the fallopian tubes leads to abdominal and low back pain, dysmenorrhea, dyspareunia, and menorrhagia. Pain is bilateral, and exacerbated by menses. _____

h. This occurs in patients that have had previous TAH-BSO and small remnants have been left behind resulting in a tender mass in the pelvis.

_____

i. An acute or chronic infection of the fallopian tubes causing cervical motion tenderness, fever, elevated WBC, and elevated ESR.

_____

j. Primarily a psychological etiology, congenital anomaly, infection, and trauma may also cause vaginal pain. _____

k. Infection of glands lying along the urethral orifice. Treatment is heat, gentle massage, and occasionally antibiotics and I&D. _____

l. Characterized by dysuria, urinary frequency, dyspareunia, and chronic inflammation of periurethral glands. Treatment of choice is pelvic floor exercises and antibiotics. _____

m. This is characterized by urinary urgency, frequency, nocturia, and severe suprapubic pain. Often there is pain on bladder filling relieved by emptying; suprapubic, pelvic, urethral, vaginal, or perineal pain; glomerulations on endoscopy or decreased compliance on cystometrograms. _____

n. Seen in athletic females with pubic and adductor muscle pain. SI joint dysfunction is also possible. Recovery is slow (7 months) and treatment should include NSAID therapy. _____

o. Indicate whether the following statements are true or false:

   i. Muscles innervated by T12-L4 can elicit visceral referral pain to the lower abdomen and rectus muscles, iliopsoas, quadratus lumborum, piriformis, and obturators.   **T or F**

   ii. Reproductive organs such as the fallopian tubes, ovaries, and the uterus are innervated by T10-L2 and can refer pain to the abdominal wall, or the pelvic floor.   **T or F**

4. Treatment of CPP:

   a. Presacral neurectomy is a procedure performed for central CPP & involves neurectomy of the _____ and _____ hypogastric plexus.   **TRUE or FALSE**

   b. What is the LUNA procedure?

   c. At which level does the epidural space end in adults? Is this different in pediatrics?

Pharmacology: Analgesic Drugs

1. Morphine:

   a. There are three subclasses of opiate receptors. Give at least one example of an agonist for each receptor indicated below:

Receptor Type	Agonist	Antagonist
Mu		Naloxone, CTOP
Delta		Naloxone, Naltrindole
Kappa		Naloxone, Nor BNI

   b. The Mu, Delta, and Kappa receptors are coupled to a protein called the "G" protein and when bound they increase _____ conduction causing the cell to hyperpolarize. This leads to a reduction in neurotransmitter release.

   c. Opiate receptors are located throughout the brain. They are most commonly found in the _____ region.

d. Binding of the Mu receptor in the PAG causes inhibition of the GABA inhibitory signal and causes excitation in the Medullospinal projections and release of NE and 5-HT.

TRUE or FALSE

e. Binding of opiates to C-fiber terminals in Rexed laminae II in the Substantia Gelatinosa causes a decrease in the Ca channel activation and release of small afferent neurotransmitters.

TRUE or FALSE

f. Binding of opiates to second order neurons (i.e. WDR neurons) increases K^+ channel permeability and leads to hyperpolarization and decreased excitability.

TRUE or FALSE

g. In the periphery, opiates can have a direct effect upon axonal conduction. These effects can be reversed by Naloxone.

TRUE or FALSE

h. Opiate central agonist activity raises the threshold to pain while peripheral activity only blocks hyperalgesia.

TRUE or FALSE

2. Non Steroidal Anti-Inflammatory Drugs (NSAIDs):

a. Peripheral injury leads to nerve terminal sensitization due to Prostaglandin synthesis via the inflammatory cascade. NSAIDs block the action of COX thereby reducing PG release.

TRUE or FALSE

b. Ketorolac and Naproxen are good analgesics but poor anti-inflammatory agents. **TRUE or FALSE**

c. COX-1 is constitutively expressed and present in kidneys and spinal cord whereas COX-2 is only constitutively expressed in platelets, & stomach. **TRUE or FALSE**

d. COX-1 expression in the periphery is inducible and takes about 3-4 hrs post stimulation to be expressed. **TRUE or FALSE**

e. Ibuprofen and Indomethacin have an equal affinity for COX-1 and COX-2. **TRUE or FALSE**

f. Repetitive C-fiber stimulation leads to spinal cord release of PGs which serves to augment the excitability of small afferents and furthers hyperalgesia. **TRUE or FALSE**

3. Spinal Alpha-2 agents:

a. Only post-synaptic alpha-2 receptors are present in the dorsal horn of the spinal cord. **TRUE or FALSE**

b. Alpha-2 receptor binding decreases Ca conductance via the CaV channels, depressing membrane excitability and pre-terminal transmitter release. **TRUE or FALSE**

c. Alpha-2 receptors are found in the Substantia Gelatinosa. **TRUE or FALSE**

4. Antidepressants:

    a. Name two antidepressants that have anti-hyperalgesic effects.

        i.

        ii.

    b. The Tricyclic Antidepressants stimulate bulbospinal pathways mediated by _____ (from Locus Coeruleus) and _____ (from Raphe Nucleus) and inhibit neurons in the dorsal horn.

5. Local Anesthetics:

    a. Sodium Channel Blockers:

        i. Sodium channel blockers perform the following functions after IV delivery: [Circle the correct statement(s)]

            1. Inhibition of axon conduction

            2. Inhibition of spontaneous activity

            3. Inhibition of neuroma firing

            4. Inhibition of DRG firing

            5. Inhibition of Glutamate evoked excitation

    b. Calcium Channel Blockers:

        i. Intrathecal Ziconotide is an N-type voltage sensitive calcium channel blocker. Where are these N-type calcium channels found?

6. Gabapentinoids:

    a. Where does Gabapentin bind? In what region of the spinal cord are the alpha-2 delta subunits expressed?

Pharmacology: Antidepressants & Anticonvulsants

1. Which of the following statements are true?

   a. Antidepressants and Anticonvulsants are effective against neuropathic pain. **T or F**

   b. Neuropathic pain describes any dysfunction of the nervous system. **T or F**

   c. The descending inhibitory systems from the brainstem onto the dorsal horn influence either a voltage gated Na channel or a voltage gated Ca channel. **T or F**

   d. Antidepressants can achieve analgesia at much lower doses than the recommended antidepressive dose. **T or F**

   e. Anticonvulsants exert their effect by stabilizing the neuronal cell membrane, decreasing neuron firing, and blocking the dorsal horn. **T or F**

2. Please categorize the following neurotransmitters as excitatory or inhibitory.

| Substance P, NMDA agonists (Glutamate), CGRP, VIP, NGF, TNFα, or CCK, Serotonin, NE, Opiates, GABA, and Glycine. ||
Excitatory	Inhibitory

3. Complete the table below which indicates some common neuropathic types of pain, the likely mechanism of action, and the preferred drug of choice.

Type of Pain	Mechanism	Drug
Burning	Peripheral sensitization, dorsal horn reorganization	
Aching	Peripheral activation of C-nociceptors	
Shooting	Ephaptic transmission	
Allodynia	Peripheral (to heat) or central (to mechanical) sensitization	
Vasomotor/ Sudomotor complaints	Sympathetic mediated	
Tinel's sign	Neuroma, nerve sprout, fascicular disruption	
Paresthesias	Dorsal horn or central neural reorganization	

4. Please specify the FDA approved indication for the medication below:

a. Duloxetine [Cymbalta]:

b. Pregabalin:

c. Topiramate, Valproic Acid:

d. Carbamazepine:

5. Please match each drug to its mechanism of action:

Drug	Mechanism of Action
a. Phenelzine, Tranylcypromine	_____ SSRI
b. Trazodone	_____ SNRI
c. Duloxetine, Venlafaxine	_____ TCA
d. Amitriptyline, Desipramine	_____ MAOI
e. Fluoxetine, Paroxetine	_____ Heterocyclics

6. What is the mechanism of action of TCA medication?

7. TCA have which of the following side effects?

        1. Anticholinergic (muscarinic, constipation)

        2. Antihistaminic (H-1 receptor block causing sedation)

        3. Anti α-1 adrenergic (orthostatic hypotension)

        4. Sexual dysfunction

        5. Some of the above (circle the correct answers)

        6. All of the above

8. Amitriptyline is metabolized to Desipramine while Nortriptyline is metabolized to Imipramine.   **TRUE or FALSE**

9. Regarding SSRI medication, Prozac has inactive metabolites and is better suited for the elderly and Zoloft has a higher protein binding and is better suited for obese patients.   **TRUE or FALSE**

10. SNRIs increase the availability of the neurotransmitters serotonin,

      _____, and _____.

11. Administration of SNRIs with the "Triptans" can precipitate a Serotonin Syndrome. Briefly describe the neurologic and cardio-respiratory consequences of this syndrome.

12. For the following agents briefly describe their mechanism of action.

    a. Carbamazepine:

b. Oxcarbazepine:

        i. Oxcarbazepine is FDA approved for which condition?

c. Gabapentin:

d. Pregabalin:

        i. This drug is FDA approved for which condition?

e. Phenytoin:

        i. Name some of the important side effects of this drug.

f. Valproic Acid:

i. Name three important side effects of this drug.

ii. This drug is FDA approved for _____.

g. Topiramate:

i. Name two important side effects of this drug.

ii. This drug is FDA approved for _____.

h. Zonisamide:

i. How is this drug different from Ziconotide?

i. Tiagabine:

j. Lamotrigine:

k. Clonazepam:

l. Levetiracetam:

m. Complete the missing data in the table below:

Drug	Channels Affected	FDA Indication
Carbamazepine		Trigeminal Neuralgia
Oxcarbazepine		Trigeminal Neuralgia
Gabapentin		
Pregabalin		PHN, Peripheral Neuropathy
Phenytoin		
Valproic Acid		Migraine prophylaxis
Topiramate		Migraine prophylaxis
Zonisamide		
Tiagabine		
Lamotrigine		
Clonazepam		
Levetiracetam		

13. Which of the following inhibit the cytochrome P3A4 enzymes?

    1. Carbamazepine, Oxcarbazepine

    2. Clarithramycin, Erythromycin

    3. Phenytoin

    4. Sertraline, Fluconazole

    5. 1 and 3 are correct

    6. 2 and 4 are correct

Pharmacology: Intraspinal Analgesics

1. Which of the following factors are important regarding access of a drug to an intraspinal receptor?

    1. Partition coefficient
    2. Density
    3. Degree of ionization
    4. Protein binding
    5. 1 and 3 are correct
    6. 2 and 4 are correct

2. Drugs with lower partition coefficients will take longer to onset and offset. They are known as hydrophobic agents. **TRUE or FALSE**

3. What are the two proposed mechanisms by which drugs placed in the epidural space enter the intrathecal space?

4. Lipophobic drugs have a delayed onset and longer duration of action. They can have a greater rostral spread leading to delayed respiratory depression.

TRUE or FALSE

5. Lipophobic drugs have a quicker onset and shorter duration of action (greater vascular uptake), and can result in greater systemic blood levels.

TRUE or FALSE

6. Lipophilic agents should be administered in the epidural space close to the site of action, whereas hydrophilic agents can be administered at any spinal level.

TRUE or FALSE

7. Intrathecal medications:
   a. Which of the following statements regarding local anesthetics are true?
      i. Bupivacaine is an ester local anesthetic   **T or F**

      ii. Bupivacaine is highly water soluble   **T or F**

      iii. Bupivacaine causes sensorimotor dissociation (blocks sensory before motor fibers)   **T or F**

      iv. Bupivacaine is cardiotoxic due to a slow diastolic dissociation constant   **T or F**

      v. Levobupivacaine has a fourfold faster dissociation constant and is much safer than Bupivacaine   **T or F**

      vi. Ropivacaine is an amide local anesthetic   **T or F**

vii.   Ropivacaine is not for use in the CSF   **T or F**

viii. Tetracaine has been shown to be neurotoxic in in-vitro models

T or F

b. What is the mechanism of action of Clonidine?

c. Clonidine works synergistically with opioids, and it has an epidural to intrathecal potency ratio of 2:1.   **TRUE or FALSE**

d. Ziconotide is a _____ channel blocker and exerts its effects at the primary afferent nociceptive fibers.

e. Ziconotide is used for neuropathic pain but it has a narrow therapeutic window.   **TRUE or FALSE**

f. Neostigmine potentiates opioid effects at the level of the spinal cord.

TRUE or FALSE

8. Intrathecal narcotic side effects:
    a. Naloxone will reverse the analgesia of lipophilic agents but not that of the hydrophilic agents (i.e. Morphine).   **TRUE or FALSE**

    b. Pruritus with intrathecal narcotics is generally due to histamine release specifically when Morphine is used.   **TRUE or FALSE**

    c.   Nalbuphine or Butorphanol both reverse the analgesia of lipophilic opioids.   **TRUE or FALSE**

9. Intrathecal Catheter Granuloma:

   a. Which of the following statements regarding an intrathecal Granuloma is correct? (circle correct answers)

      i. A Granuloma is a fibrotic mass that occurs where intrathecal catheters are placed

      ii. It can occur due to increased drug concentration (Morphine 50mg/ml)

      iii. It can occur due to increased duration of infusion (> 25mg Morphine/24hrs)

      iv. It commonly occurs when the dose of Morphine exceeds 10mg/24hrs

      v. Granuloma formation can also occur with Clonidine

   b. What is the proposed mechanism of Granuloma formation?

   c. Will cessation of intrathecal infusions result in resolution of a Granuloma? If so, how long does it take for the Granuloma to resolve?

   d. When should the patient be taken to the operating room for a surgical removal of the catheter?

Chapter 27

Pharmacology: NSAIDs

1. Review the biochemical pathway of NSAIDs below:

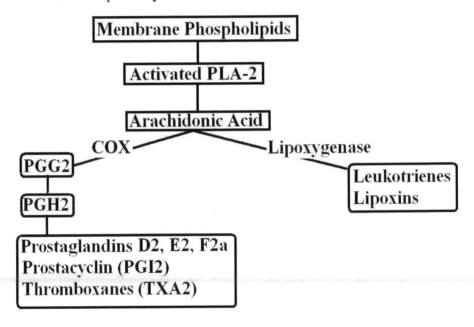

2. Corticosteroids inhibit _____, while NSAIDs and ASA
   inhibit _____.

3. Why is NSAID use contraindicated in patients with Asthma?

4. What is the triad of Samter's syndrome?

5. Match the physiologic function below with either the COX-1 or COX-2 enzyme.

  - PGI-2 production (Gastric protection)   _____
  - Pro-inflammatory PGs   _____
  - PGE2 production (Renal function)   _____
  - Inflammatory mediators   _____
  - TXA2 production (platelet function)   _____

6. COX-1 is an inducible enzyme found in normal cells while COX-2 is a constitutive enzyme found in inflammatory cells.   **TRUE or FALSE**

7. The central mechanism for NSAID mediated analgesic effects relies on prostaglandin formation due to central sensitization. **TRUE or FALSE**

8. Intrathecal NSAIDs reduce hyperalgesia by affecting the actions of substance P, activating serotonergic descending pathways, down regulating NMDA receptor sites, and modulating Glutamate synthesis. **TRUE or FALSE**

9. The Sulfonamides (i.e. Celebrex) should not be used in patients with a "Sulfa allergy".   **TRUE or FALSE**

10. The "older" COX-2 inhibitors which were not marketed as COX-2 blockers include _____, and _____.

11. The NSAID family is composed of Carboxylic acids, Pyrazoles, Oxicams, and the Coxibs. On the next page, provide an example for each NSAID family.

a. Carboxylic acids:

    i. Salicylic Acids   <u>Aspirin</u>_____

    ii. Acetic Acids   _____

    iii. Propionic Acids   _____

    iv. Anthranilic Acids _____

b. Pyrazoles   _____

c. Oxicams   _____

d. Coxibs   _____

12. Which of the following NSAIDs are inactive prodrugs that require biotransformation to become active?

    1. Etodolac

    2. Dolobid

    3. Nabumetone

    4. Naproxen

    5. 1 and 3 are correct

    6. 2 and 4 are correct

    7. All are correct

13. The adverse effects associated with NSAID use are due to their ability to inhibit prostaglandin synthesis.   **TRUE or FALSE**

14. Regarding NSAID related complications, fill in the blanks, state whether the statement is true or false, and answer the following questions.

    a. NSAIDs inhibit _____ synthesis and reduce gastric cytoprotection.

b. Two important predisposing factors that can lead to NSAID gastropathy include _____ , and _____ .

c. Treatment for gastropathy can include Misoprostol. Why is this drug contraindicated in pregnancy?

d. ASA causes reversible inhibition of COX leading to platelet dysfunction for the life of platelets (6-10 days).

TRUE or FALSE

e. All other NSAIDs cause an irreversible inhibition of COX leading to normal hemostasis after 5 (drug) half lives. **TRUE or FALSE**

f. NSAIDs block PGI-2 synthesis therefore inhibiting platelet aggregation, while Coxibs prevent TXA-2 synthesis allowing for normal platelet aggregation.   **TRUE or FALSE**

g. In stress states, PGs induce renal vasodilatation leading to increased renal blood flow.   **TRUE or FALSE**

h. NSAIDs can lead to increased BP, CHF, edema, hyperkalemia, and acute renal failure.   **TRUE or FALSE**

i. NSAIDs cause the production of histologically and biomechanically inferior bone.   **TRUE or FALSE**

j. Explain the proposed mechanism of COX-2 related cerebrovascular and thrombotic events.

Pharmacology: Opioids

1. Opiates are agents that have analgesic properties, while Opioids are derived from opium. **TRUE or FALSE**

2. The only two drugs that are derived from the poppy plant include _____ and _____.

3. Opioid receptors serve two functions; the "binding affinity" correlates with analgesic potency while the molecular recognition correlates with analgesic activity. **TRUE or FALSE**

4. Only narcotic L-isomers exhibit analgesic activity. **TRUE or FALSE**

5. Rank the following compounds in order of binding affinity (1=high, 5= low):

Opioid	Binding Affinity
Alfentanil	
Meperidine	
Fentanyl	
Morphine	
Sufentanil	

6. Which Mu receptor is mostly responsible for the negative side effects of narcotics?

7. Opioids bind the same receptors as the endogenous opioids our bodies produce such as the _____, the _____, and the _____.

8. Concomitant administration of an opioid partial and a full agonist reduces (antagonizes) the effect of the full agonist.   **TRUE or FALSE**

9. Opioid receptor partial antagonists inhibit binding to a single opioid receptor type while full antagonists prevent opioid binding at all receptor sites.

    TRUE or FALSE

10. Opioid mixed agonist-antagonists have divergent activities at different receptors.   **TRUE or FALSE**

11. Provide at least two examples of opioid mixed agonist-antagonists.
    a.
    b.

12. Write at least one characteristic feature for each medication listed below:
    a. Butorphanol

    b. Nalbuphine

    c. Buprenorphine

13. Specific Opiates and Opioids:

    a. Morphine has two active metabolites. What are they and which one is the active metabolite?

    b. Morphine metabolites are cleared in the kidneys. Which of the following narcotics would be considered safe in a patient with renal failure? (circle the correct answer)

        i. Hydromorphone

        ii. Fentanyl

        iii. Hydrocodone

        iv. Oxymorphone

        v. Meperidine

    c. What aspect of codeine metabolism relates to its analgesic effect?

    d. Dextromethorphan is the L-isomer of Morphine and is useful for neuropathic pain.   **TRUE or FALSE**

    e. Approximately 1/3 of any Oxycontin dose is released during the first hour; the remaining 2/3 is released as the long acting form.

          TRUE or FALSE

    f. Morphine's D-isomer (Dextromethorphan) is methylated to a metabolite called Dextrophan which is Levorphanol's D-isomer.

          TRUE or FALSE

g. Methadone has a primary half life of 14 hours and a secondary half life of 55 hours. Its slow terminal elimination leads to an analgesic duration that is much shorter than the half life.

TRUE or FALSE

h. The D-isomer of Methadone is a _____ receptor antagonist. It also inhibits 5-HT and NE reuptake.

TRUE or FALSE

i. Meperidine's active metabolite is called _____. Meperidine is contraindicated in patients on MAOIs because its metabolite can lead to CNS excitation.

TRUE or FALSE

j. The only D-isomer that has traditional analgesic properties is called

_____.

k. Complete the missing information in the table below which illustrates the equianalgesic dose of some common narcotics.

Opioid	IV	Oral
Morphine	10	30
Hydromorphone		
Meperidine		
Methadone	N/A	
Oxycodone ≈ Hydrocodone	N/A	
Codeine	N/A	
Fentanyl		

l. Complete the table below which shows equianalgesic doses of morphine:

IV	Epidural	Subarachnoid	ICV
10			

m. Can Narcan reverse seizures caused by high doses of narcotics? Can Narcan reverse seizures caused by Normeperidine?

n. Please indicate the schedule classification (class I through V) for each item below:

     i. Heroin   _____

     ii. Promethazine   _____

     iii. Hydrocodone with Tylenol   _____

     iv. Lorazepam   _____

     v. Buprenorphine   _____

     vi. Morphine   _____

     vii. Codeine with Tylenol   _____

     viii. Codeine   _____

     ix. Hydrocodone   _____

     x. Marijuana   _____

o. Naloxone blocks two types of opioid receptors. Please name the two receptors and indicate the physiologic function of each receptor.

     i.

     ii.

p. The duration of action of a single dose of Naloxone is 120 minutes.

TRUE or FALSE

q. Name two critical side effects of opioid reversal with Narcan.

    i.

    ii.

r. Flumazenil and Naloxone have the same duration of action.

TRUE or FALSE

s. The ideal body weight should be utilized to determine the appropriate dosage of a particular lipid soluble drug.

TRUE or FALSE

Pharmacology: Steroids

1. The antero-lateral and postero-lateral annulus of a disk is innervated by

   _____. The outer 1/3 to ½ of the lateral annulus is

   innervated by _____, and the posterior annulus, anterior

   dural sac and dural sleeve are innervated by the

   _____.

2. Which of the following statements regarding discogenic pain are true?

   i. Discogenic pain is radicular in nature

   ii. Discogenic pain can be exacerbated by sneezing or coughing

   iii. 75 % of patients with discogenic pain have a spontaneous
       resolution of symptoms within one year

   iv. 1 and 3 are correct

   v. All are correct

   vi. Only one of the above is correct (circle the answer)

3. State at least two surgical indications for a patient presenting with a herniated
   nucleus pulposus.

4. How do steroids decrease and inhibit the inflammatory response? How do steroids exert their anti-nociceptive effects?

5. The only truly non-particulate steroid is _____, followed by _____ which is minimally particulate containing.

6. The most potent steroid on a mg/ml basis is _____.

7. Polyethylene glycol which is present in some of the steroid preparations (at a 2.86% concentration) has been implicated in causing what condition?

8. What are some complications associated with intrathecal injection of steroids?

9. The following steroids are organized from least to most potent. State the common epidural dose, and indicate the equipotent dose in the table below:

Steroid	Common Epidural Dose	Glucocorticoid Equipotent Dose (mg)
Cortisone, Hydrocortisone	N/A	
Prednisone, Prednisolone	N/A	
Methylprednisolone		
Triamcinolone		
Dexamethasone		
Betamethasone		1

Psychogenic Pain

1. Mood Disorders (Axis I):

    a. Mood disorders

        i. Major depressive disorder (MDD) is defined by _____ weeks of depression or loss of interest accompanied by at least _____ additional symptoms (SIGECAPS).

        ii. The incidence of depression in patients with chronic pain can range from 50-100%! **TRUE or FALSE**

        iii. Manic disorder is defined as an abnormal and persistent elevated or expressive or irritable mood lasting _____ days or more with three or more additional symptoms.

        iv. Hypomanic disorder is characterized by an elevated, expansive, and irritable mood lasting ____ days or more with three or more additional symptoms.

        v. Hypomanic individuals may not require hospitalization, but can presents with psychotic features. **TRUE or FALSE**

vi. Two years of numerous periods of hypomanic symptoms that do not meet the criteria for a manic episode and numerous periods of depression symptoms that do not meet criteria for major depressive disorder is characteristic of _____ disorder.

vii. What is Dysthymic disorder?

viii. How is Bipolar I different from Bipolar II disorder?

b. Provide a diagnosis for each of the following descriptions using the list below. [Agoraphobia, OCD, PTSD, Panic attack, Acute stress disorder, Generalized anxiety disorder]

i. Obsessions (thoughts) causing marked anxiety or distress and or compulsions (behaviors) which serve to neutralize the anxiety. _____

ii. Sudden onset of intense apprehension, fear, or terror associated with feelings of impending doom, SOB, palpitations, or chest pain. _____

iii. Re-experiencing of an extremely traumatic event accompanied by symptoms of increased arousal and avoidance of stimuli associated with the trauma. _____

iv. PTSD type symptoms occurring immediately after a traumatic event.

_____

v. At least 6 months of persistent and excessive anxiety. Generalized anxiety disorder is present in 28-63% of patients with chronic pain.

_____

vi. Fear, anxiety, avoidance of situations or places where escape may be difficult or help not available.

_____

2. Personality Disorders (Axis II):

a. Match the descriptions with the correct Personality Cluster type (A, B, or C):

i. This cluster describes the odd, eccentric personalities (paranoid, schizoid).   Cluster _____

ii. This cluster describes the dramatic or manipulative personalities (histrionic, borderline, & antisocial).

Cluster _____

iii. This cluster describes the anxious personalities (dependent, obsessive compulsive).   Cluster _____

3. Provide a diagnosis for each of the following descriptions using the list below. [Paranoid, Schizoid, Schizotypal, Borderline, Anti-social, Histrionic, Narcissistic, Avoidant, Dependent, Obsessive Compulsive]

a. Submissive and clinging behavior related to an excessive need to be taken care of. _____

b. A pattern of distrust and suspiciousness such that other's motives are interpreted as malevolent. _____

c. A pattern of instability in interpersonal relationships, self image and affects, and marked impulsivity. _____

d. Excessive emotionality & attention seeking. _____

e. Pre-occupation with orderliness, perfection, and control.

_____

f. Grandiosity, need for admiration, and lack of empathy.

_____

g. Detachment from social relationships and restricted range of emotional expression. _____

h. A pattern of acute discomfort in close relationships, cognitive or perceptual distortions, and egocentric behavior. _____

i. A pattern of disregard for and violation of the rights of others.

_____

j. A pattern of social inhibition, feelings of inadequacy, and hypersensitivity to negative evaluation. _____

4. In _____ disorder the symptoms are not intentional and cause clinical impairment or distress in social and occupational circumstances.

5. In _____ disorder there is unexplained symptoms or deficits, affecting sensory or motor function that suggests a neurological or other general medical condition but do not conform to known anatomical pathways.

6. This disorder is characterized by a preoccupation with the fear or idea of having a serious disease based on one's misinterpretation of bodily symptoms. This disorder is called _____.

7. In Somatoform disorder patients fabricate symptoms that are self inflicted, exaggerated, and intentional.   **TRUE or FALSE**

8. Factitious disorder is much like Somatoform disorder in that there is a psychological need to assume the sick role.   **TRUE or FALSE**

9. Factitious disorder is much like Malingering in that patients are motivated by external incentives and have something to gain by their "disease".

                    TRUE or FALSE

10. Match the related substance disorder with its definition:

a. Substance Dependence   ____A primary, chronic, neurobiological disease characterized by behaviors (3 Cs)

b. Addiction   ____A patient conditioned to behave like an addict due to multiple failed treatments

c. Substance Abuse   ____A state of adaptation manifested by a withdrawal syndrome

d. Pseudo-addiction   ____Illicit arrangements intended to result in the physical delivery of controlled drugs for non-prescribed uses

e. Diversion   ____The misuse of a drug for recreational reasons

11. List at least four methods that can be utilized to identify and reject a potential drug abusing patient.

     a.

     b.

     c.

     d.

12. Is there a relationship between lower pain threshold and lack of sleep? Explain.

Psychologic Assessment of Pain

1. Assessment tools:

    a. What type of information does the McGill-Melzack Pain questionnaire provide?

    b. Minnesota Multiphasic Personality Inventory is one of the best predictors of pain and _____ outcome following _____.

    c. Beck Depression Inventory evaluates the presence of depression in chronic pain patients; what components of pain are specifically evaluated using this test?

2. Assign the tests in the following list to the correct description: [Pain Disability Index, Oswestry Pain Scale, Brief Pain Inventory]

    a. This test assesses pain at different times (highest, lowest, & average) and its level of interference on ADLs. _____

b. This test evaluates a patient's perception of the severity of disability in one's functional status due to pain.   _____

c. This test evaluates pain intensity, disability and level of functionality.

_____

3. Match the tests to the correct description:

a. Chronic Pain Acceptance Questionnaire

____ Evaluates exaggerated negative orientation toward a noxious stimulus

b. Coping Strategies Questionnaire

____ Evaluates level of disengagement from pain, and a realistic appraisal of appropriate expectations and engagement in positive every day activities.

c. Pain Catastrophizing Scale

____ Assesses what patients do and how they cope with their chronic pain.

d. Chronic Pain Coping Inventory

____ Evaluates various strategies used by patients to cope with their pain.

4. Which of the following risk factors are associated with the presence of pain either early or later in life?

    1. Physical or sexual abuse

    2. Love and support received due to presence of pain

    3. Parental Abandonment or emotional neglect

    4. Alcohol or drug abuse as a teenager

    5. 1 and 3 are correct

    6. 2 and 4 are correct

5. Pain and pain relief can be best measured via:

    1. The use of pain scales, and questionnaires

    2. Reduction in analgesics consumption

    3. Functional ability outcomes

    4. Pain reduction of 20% or greater

    5. All of the above

Psychological Treatment of Pain

1. Examples of behavioral therapies include: (circle the correct answers)

    a. Relaxation

    b. Biofeedback

    c. Operant conditioning

    d. Exposure/desensitization. escape or avoidance

    e. Classical conditioning

2. Which of the following cognitive factors affect pain perception:

    a. Pain appraisal

    b. Beliefs about pain

    c. Coping

    d. Self efficacy

    e. A and C are correct

    f. B and D are correct

    g. All are correct

3. Give two examples of psychological therapies employed in the treatment of pain.

Radiologic Approaches to Pain Medicine

1. Techniques related to spine imaging:

    a. What advantage(s) do X-rays have over CT imaging of bones and joints?

    b. On X-ray, subluxation of up to _____mm on flexion/extension films is considered normal.

    c. The Atlanto-Dental Interval (ADI) is the space between the

       _____ and _____. This space is

       widened in patients with _____.

    d. Facet disease and neuroforaminal narrowing due to osseous

       obstruction can be evaluated via _____ views for the

       cervical region and _____ views for the lumbar region.

    e. CT is mainly used for the evaluation of bone and soft tissue.

                                                         TRUE or FALSE

f. CT scanning allows for excellent evaluation of C1 and C2 specifically in evaluation of fractures. **TRUE or FALSE**

g. CT scanning helps determine uncovertebral disease which is found in the joint space from _____. **TRUE or FALSE**

h. MRI is invaluable for the evaluation of subtle endplate or vertebral body fractures, edema, and articular facet capsule injury.

TRUE or FALSE

i. MRI is used for the evaluation of soft tissue, bone marrow, infection, inflammation, and tumors. **TRUE or FALSE**

j. Match the following MRI imaging technique to the correct description.

a. T2   ___ Used to identify infection and tumor. Gadolinium is hyper-intense in T1 weighted images as is fat. Hence a fat suppressed T1 Gad image will identify regions of inflammation, infection, or tumor.

b. STIR   ___ Excellent for fluid evaluation. Tumors and edema will appear hyper-intense in these images.

c. T1 with fat saturation post-gadolinium   ___ This is a specialized T2 weighted image sequence with fat suppression. CSF, edema, and tumors will be hyper-intense in these images.

d. T1   ___ This is a T2 weighted image that hyper-intensifies blood and is used to evaluate blood in the spinal cord or other regions.

e. GRE   ___ Excellent for evaluation of anatomy and fat. Fat will appear hyper-intense (bright) in these images. Hypo-intense signals are demonstrated by air, water, and sclerosis.

2. Pain producing pathologies:

    a. The nucleus pulposus appears dark on T2 images while the annulus fibrosis appears bright on T2 images.   **TRUE or FALSE**

    b. Transverse disc tears cause pain but they do not appear hyper-intense on T2 images.   **TRUE or FALSE**

    c. Radial disc tears produce pain and are hyper-intense on T2 images.   **TRUE or FALSE**

    d. In the cervical region, a central herniation at C3-4 will affect the _____ nerve root whereas a foraminal herniation at the same level will affect the _____ nerve root.

    e. In the lumbar region, a central herniation at L3-4 will affect the _____ nerve root whereas a foraminal herniation at the same level will affect the _____ nerve root.

    f. What are Modic changes? Distinguish between Modic 1, 2, and 3.

    g. Spondylolysis is thought to be due to microtrauma & is characterized by a _____ in the pars intra-articularis.

    h. Spondylolysis may present with Spondylolisthesis without central spinal stenosis.   **TRUE or FALSE**

Regional Anesthesia: Upper & Lower Extremity

1. Upper extremity:

   a. An Axillary block is best utilized for pain in what region of the upper extremity?

   b. A successful Axillary block will inhibit the flexors of the upper extremity first.   **TRUE or FALSE**

   c. An Infraclavicular block can be utilized for surgery on which portion of the upper extremity?

   d. The risk of pneumothorax is highest with the Infraclavicular block.

   TRUE or FALSE

   e. Acceptable twitches for this block include that of the pectoralis major, biceps, or the deltoid   **TRUE or FALSE**

   f. A Supraclavicular block is utilized for pain distal to the _____.

   TRUE or FALSE

g. The Phrenic nerve is blocked 100% of the time with this block and 50% of the time with Supraclavicular blocks. What block is this?

h. The Suprascapular nerve is sensory to the deltoid muscle and can result in a failed block if relying on the paresthesia technique alone.

   TRUE or FALSE

i. In the cervical region, the distance from skin to the vertebral body is approximately _____ cm, and to the spinal cord is _____ cm.

j. There is a greater propensity to block the entire sympathetic outflow to an extremity with a regional technique than with an isolated sympathetic technique.

   TRUE or FALSE

k. Name at least 3 side effects and complications of upper extremity blocks.

2. Lower extremity:
   a. The lower extremity is supplied by 3 nerves from the lumbar plexus, and 2 nerves from the sacral plexus. Name these nerves.

b. When performing a sciatic nerve block which of the following responses are most favorable?

     1. Plantar flexion

     2. Dorsiflexion

     3. Inversion

     4. Eversion

     5. 1 and 3

     6. 2 and 4

c. Which nerve roots does the femoral nerve originate from?

d. The deep division of the femoral nerve provides sensory innervation to which region of the body?

e. The foot is supplied by 4 terminal branches of the sciatic nerve, and one terminal branch of the femoral nerve. Name these nerves and indicate their location on the image below.

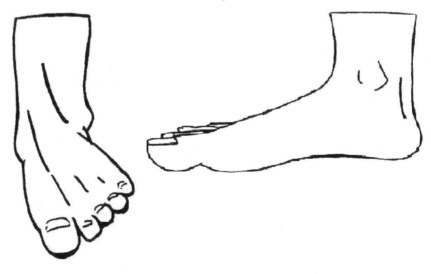

3. Match the following terms to the correct description of nerve injury:
[Neuropraxia, Axonotmesis, Neurotmesis]

    a. This occurs when the axons and the Schwann cells are disrupted. This is the most severe type of nerve injury and is called

        _____.

    b. When the nerve is intact after injury but does not transmit impulses it is called _____. It is usually transient and occurs due to compression.

    c. When the axon is severed, the Schwann sheath remains intact and so this injury usually heals. This is called _____.

    d. After nerve injury, the distal segment of the nerve degenerates. Regeneration can occur at a rate of _____ mm/day.

    e. If no re-innervation occurs by one year following nerve injury, then no further healing will occur and the denervated muscle fibers begin to disintegrate & atrophy.   **TRUE or FALSE**

    f. It takes 7-10 days for paraspinal muscles, and 14-21 days for distal extremity muscles to show signs of fibrillation after nerve injury. This is when NCV and EMG testing should be performed to determine the presence of prior myoneural injury.   **TRUE or FALSE**

Rehabilitation Medicine

1. Patients lean away from a painful joint when walking (antalgia) and lean towards a side or muscle that is weak.   **TRUE or FALSE**

2. Assistive devices decrease the weight experienced by the patient and allow for greater mobility. Canes decrease weight by _____ %, crutches decrease weight by _____ %, and walkers decrease weight by _____ %.

3. Based on the following descriptions, determine the correct rehabilitation or physical therapy modality using the following list:

   [Heat, Cold, Water, Topical medication, Traction, Massage, Manipulation, Exercise, Orthotics, Electrotherapy]

   a. _____ increases pliability of collagen, decreases joint stiffness, resolves inflammatory reaction, increases blood flow, & decreases peristalsis.

   b. _____ provide sensory stimulation and pain relief. One can utilize rubifacients made of capsaicin/menthol, creams, ointments, phonophoresis, iontophoresis, and injections.

c. _____ can provide pressure massage, hot soaks, steam baths for relaxation or to "shock" and restart the sympathetic nervous system.

d. _____ controls bleeding, induces vaso-constriction, controls spasm, & reduces inflammatory reactions.

e. _____ used to prevent or correct a deformity, improve function, and relieve pain.

f. _____ feels great, removes metabolic wastes, decreases edema, stretches soft tissue, stimulates blood flow, mobilizes scar tissue, and reduces stretch.

g. _____ restores anatomic alignment, decreases nerve and muscle compression, and loosens stiff muscle attachments.

h. _____ uses electric modalities to achieve pharmaceutical and biologic effects by affecting the voltage gated ion channels on cell membranes causing them to open and resulting in a nodal block.

i. _____ provides stretch to soft tissue, provides joint distraction, enlarges foramen or disc space, decompresses nerve, can be static or dynamic, and provides segmental treatment.

j. _____ maintains mobility, range of motion, neuromuscular coordination, posture recovery, strength gain, increases endurance, and helps to decrease pain.

4. Cold laser therapy is FDA approved for which conditions?

    a. Carpal tunnel pain

    b. Neck and shoulder pain

    c. Arthritis pain

    d. Joint pain

    e. Muscle spasm

    f. A and C are correct

    g. B and D are correct

    h. Only one answer is correct

    i. All are correct

5. Which of the following characterize the therapeutic effects of electrical therapy?

    a. Reduction of edema at an injury site

    b. Neuroprobing

    c. Electrogalvanic stimulation

    d. Interferential therapy

    e. A and C are correct

    f. B and D are correct

    g. All are correct

6. Electrotherapy is base on the gate control theory. Describe this theory.

Spinal and Epidural Anesthesia

1. In adults, the spinal cord ends at which spinal level?

    At which level does the dura end?

    At which level does the epidural space end?

    Are these levels different in children, if so how?

2. What is Tuffier's line and what is its significance?

3. Indicate the surface anatomy landmark for each item below:

      i. C7: _____

     ii. T7: _____

   iii. L1: _____

   iv. L4: _____

     v. S2: _____

4. Where are the vertebral arteries located and how far do they extend?

5. What is the artery of Adamkiewicz? What region does it supply? (be as specific as possible)

6. Infarction of the anterior spinal artery leads to _____.

7. Where is CSF formed? Describe the path of CSF using terms such as "Monro", "Luschka", "Sylvius", and "Megendie".

8. Describe the theorized etiology of Post Dural Puncture Headache. What are some common symptoms and how is it treated.

9. Which of the following factors affect the spread of local anesthetic in the subarachnoid space?
   a. Baricity
   b. Barbotage
   c. Patient position
   d. Speed of injection
   e. A and C are correct
   f. B and D are correct
   g. All are correct

10. Which of the following factors affects the duration of spinal anesthesia?
    a. Drug used
    b. Spread achieved
    c. Dose injected
    d. Age and general condition of the patient
    e. A and C are correct
    f. B and D are correct
    g. All are correct

11. The addition of epinephrine to Lidocaine or Bupivacaine will increase their duration of action in the intrathecal space.   **TRUE or FALSE**

12. Define Decremental Conduction.

13. While opioids work primarily in the Substantia Gelatinosa, local anesthetics work in Laminae I, III, and V of the dorsal root entry zone.

TRUE or FALSE

14. How does the presentation of an epidural abscess compare to that of an epidural hematoma?

15. How does anterior spinal artery syndrome present? Is it reversible?

16. What is the etiology behind adhesive arachnoiditis? How many days until the onset of symptoms?

17. Describe at least three signs or symptoms of CNS local anesthetic toxicity.

18. Hypotension and bradycardia can occur after spinal anesthetics due to

_____ block which affects the heart rate, venous

return, and contractility.

19. The GI system receives both sympathetic and parasympathetic innervation.

TRUE or FALSE

20. Prilocaine and Benzocaine toxicity can lead to a hematologic condition called

_____.

21. Prilocaine has a metabolite called _____ which can

lead to central cyanosis. The condition created can be treated with Methylene

Blue 1 mg/kg.

Chapter 37

Sympathetic Nervous System Pain

1. General anatomy:

    a. The parasympathetic nervous system (PNS) is called the Cranio-Sacral nervous system and includes cranial nerves ____, ____, ____, ____, and nerve roots _____.

    b. The sympathetic nervous system (SNS) is called the Thoraco-Lumbar nervous system and includes spinal nerves from _____.

    c. The preganglionic neurons send axons to the para-vertebral chain as _____ rami communicantes. Once these fibers enter the para-vertebral ganglion, they can synapse at the level entered, or they can ascend or descend to a different level. These rami may also pass through and synapse onto a post ganglionic neuron called a _____ ganglion.

    d. The Postganglionic fibers are unmyelinated and are referred to as _____ rami communicantes.

e. Splanchnic nerves are preganglionic sympathetic fibers in the thoraco-lumbar region and parasympathetic in the pelvic region.

TRUE or FALSE

f. The superior and middle hypogastric plexuses are sympathetic ganglions while the inferior hypogastric plexus carries both parasympathetic and sympathetic nerve fibers.

TRUE or FALSE

g. The Stellate ganglion is the confluence of the superior thoracic and the first cervical ganglion.   **TRUE or FALSE**

h. The Stellate ganglion blocks sympathetic outflow from the middle cervical to T4 or T5.   **TRUE or FALSE**

i. Sympathetic blocks are performed at the site of synapse and not at the origin of the pre-ganglionic fibers.   **TRUE or FALSE**

j. Complete the missing information in the table below:

Structure	Origin of Pre-ganglionic Fiber	Site of synapse	Route of post-gang. Fiber
Head and neck	T1-T2		Internal and external carotid plexus
Upper extremity	T2-T8		Gray rami to brachial plexus
Lower extremity	T10-L2		Gray rami to lumbar and lumbo-sacral plexus
Abdomen	T5-T11		Gastric, pancreatic plexus

k. Local anesthetic sympathetic blocks are used for:

     1. Acute pancreatitis

     2. Myocardial infarction

     3. Ruptured peptic ulcer

     4. Renal or biliary colic

     5. I don't know! I'll just circle the correct answer.

l. A volume as much as _____ cc in the vertebral artery can result in systemic toxicity and seizures.

m. Successful sympathetic denervation of the head and neck involves blocking of the _____ ganglion. The block is performed at the level of C6 also called _____.

n. What is Horner's syndrome, what does it indicate?

o. State at least three complications of a stellate ganglion block.

p. The greater splanchnic nerve is found at the _____ level.

q. The greater, lesser, and least splanchnics are pre-vertebral structures whereas the celiac plexus is a para-vertebral structure.

                                                                 TRUE or FALSE

r. The nerves of the celiac plexus originate from _____. The celiac plexus is formed anterior to the aorta at the level of _____. The celiac plexus block is performed in the _____-crural space.

s. Complications of a celiac plexus block include:

    1. Backache

    2. Severe orthostatic hypotension

    3. Lumbar plexus block

    4. Unopposed parasympathetics

    5. Circle the most likely answer(s)

t. Seventy five percent of the blood supply to spinal cord is derived from the _____ which arises from the vertebral artery caudal to the basilar artery.

u. Arteria Radicularis Magna most commonly arises at _____ on the left side and supplies what part of the spinal cord?

v. The lumbar plexus is a para-vertebral structure and is composed of four pairs of ganglia from _____ to _____.

w. Genitofemoral neuralgia is a complications of lumbar plexus block due to injection into the _____.

x. Intravenous regional anesthesia only blocks the efferent sympathetic fibers.   **TRUE or FALSE**

y. Guanethidine has a postganglionic site of action. Please describe the mechanism of action of this drug.

z. Concurrent use of Guanethidine should be avoided with which class of medications?

2. A schematic of the Sympathetic and the Parasympathetic nervous system is illustrated in the following pages. Please review and commit to memory.

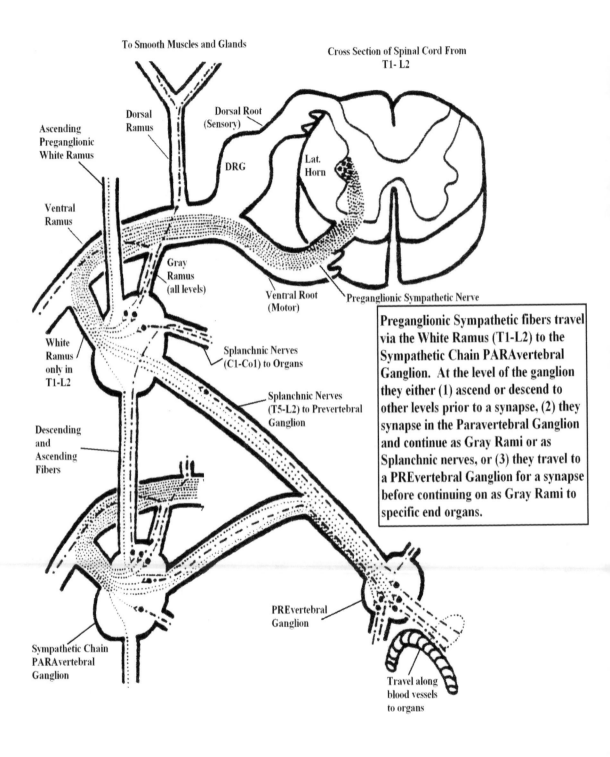

To Smooth Muscles and Glands

Cross Section of Spinal Cord From
T1- L2

Dorsal
Ramus

Dorsal Root
(Sensory)

Ascending
Preganglionic
White Ramus

DRG

Lat.
Horn

Ventral
Ramus

Gray
Ramus
(all levels)

Ventral Root
(Motor)

Preganglionic Sympathetic Nerve

White
Ramus
only in
T1-L2

Splanchnic Nerves
(C1-Co1) to Organs

Splanchnic Nerves
(T5-L2) to Prevertebral
Ganglion

Descending
and
Ascending
Fibers

Preganglionic Sympathetic fibers travel
via the White Ramus (T1-L2) to the
Sympathetic Chain PARAvertebral
Ganglion. At the level of the ganglion
they either (1) ascend or descend to
other levels prior to a synapse, (2) they
synapse in the Paravertebral Ganglion
and continue as Gray Rami or as
Splanchnic nerves, or (3) they travel to
a PREvertebral Ganglion for a synapse
before continuing on as Gray Rami to
specific end organs.

PREvertebral
Ganglion

Sympathetic Chain
PARAvertebral
Ganglion

Travel along
blood vessels
to organs

········· Preganglionic Sympathetic

·—·—·— Postganglioni Sympathetic

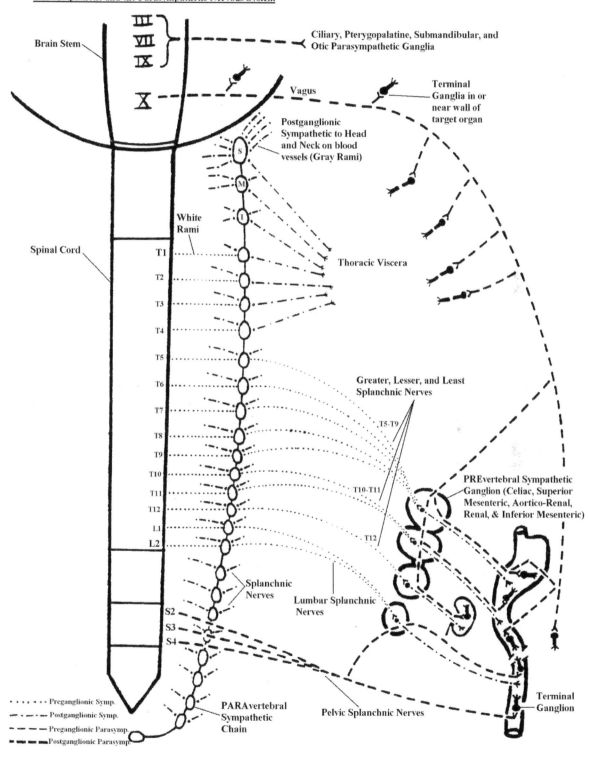

The Sympathetic and the Parasympathetic Nervous System

Brain Stem

Ciliary, Pterygopalatine, Submandibular, and Otic Parasympathetic Ganglia

Vagus

Terminal Ganglia in or near wall of target organ

Postganglionic Sympathetic to Head and Neck on blood vessels (Gray Rami)

White Rami

Spinal Cord

Thoracic Viscera

Greater, Lesser, and Least Splanchnic Nerves

T5-T9

T10-T11

PREvertebral Sympathetic Ganglion (Celiac, Superior Mesenteric, Aortico-Renal, Renal, & Inferior Mesenteric)

T12

Splanchnic Nerves

Lumbar Splanchnic Nerves

Terminal Ganglion

PARAvertebral Sympathetic Chain

Pelvic Splanchnic Nerves

· · · · · · · Preganglionic Symp.
— · — · — · Postganglionic Symp.
— — — — Preganglionic Parasymp.
▬ ▬ ▬ ▬ Postganglionic Parasymp.

Trauma Pain

1. Post traumatic or post Surgical:

   a. Rib fracture associated injuries can cause damage to which nerve resulting in winged scapulae?

   b. When performing an intercostal nerve block, how are the vein, artery, and nerve arranged relative to the rib?

   c. A clavicular fracture can result in injury to which bundle of nerves?

   d. Describe the mechanism of action of subarachnoid opioids. Describe which receptors are blocked and in which region of the spinal cord they exert their effect.

   e. Latency of onset of effect in intrathecal opioid administration is directly related to the drug's _____.

f. How does intrathecal Morphine cause urinary retention?

g. Onset of respiratory depression for any narcotic is based on its
    hydrophobicity.   **TRUE or FALSE**

h. The only opioid with local anesthetic properties is _____.

i. The analgesic mechanism of action of Clonidine is such that it inhibits
    _____ release and acts as an alpha-2 agonist.

j. Complete the missing information regarding intrathecal opioids in the
    table below:

Opioid	Typical dose	Latency	Duration of Analgesia
Morphine			480-1440 min
Meperidine			60-400 min
Fentanyl			30-120 min
Sufentanil			60-180 min

k. With respect to epidural analgesia the "Dural Transport" theory states
    that the terminal and functional elimination half life of an opioid in the
    lumbar epidural space is related to its _____, whereas in
    the thoracic space it is based on its _____.

l. For hydrophilic opioids, analgesia is independent of catheter
    congruency to surgical site.   **TRUE or FALSE**

m. The narcotic effects of epidural morphine is negatively affected by local anesthetics such as 2-Chlorprocaine.   **TRUE or FALSE**

n. As an adjunctive epidural medication, Ketamine is only effective if added to morphine.   **TRUE or FALSE**

o. Complete the missing information regarding epidural opioids in the table below:

Opioid	Single dose	Onset (min)	Duration (hrs)	Infusion (mcg/ml)	Infusion rate
Morphine				10	0.1-1 (mg/hr)
Hydromorphone				5-10	0.1-0.2 (mg/hr)
Methadone				10-15	0.3-0.5 (mg/hr)
Meperidine				2500	10-30 (mcg/hr)
Sufentanil				1	10-20 (mcg/hr)
Fentanyl				5-10	25-100 (mcg/hr)

p. Indicate the level of epidural catheter placement for each region listed below:

    i. Thoracic: _____

    ii. Upper Abdominal: _____

    iii. Lower Abdominal: _____

    iv. Hip: _____

    v. Knee: _____

    vi. Perineum: _____

References

Ballantyne, J., Fishman, S., & Abdi, S. (2002). The Massachusetts General Hospital Handbook of Pain Management. Philadelphia: Lippincott Williams & Wilkins.

Benzon, H., Raja, S., Molloy, R., Liu, S., & Fishman, S. (2005). Essentials of Pain Medicine and Regional Anesthesia. Philadelphia: Churchill Livingstone.

Brown, D. (1999). Atlas of Regional Anesthesia. Philadelphia: Saunders.

Chelly, J. (2004). Peripheral Nerve Blocks: A Color Atlas. Philadelphia: Lippincott Williams & Wilkins.

Cousins, M., Bridenbaugh, P. (1988). Neural Blockade: In Clinical Anesthesia and Management of Pain. Philadelphia: J. B. Lippincott Company.

Dannemiller Memorial Education Foundation (2007). An Intensive Review of the Specialty of Pain Medicine (Power Point Slides). Web site: http://www.dannemiller.com.

Fonda, B., Ezerman, E. (1997). Human Gross Anatomy. Burlington: University of Vermont.

Greenberg, D., Aminoff, M., & Simon, R. (1993). Clinical Neurology. Norwalk: Appleton & Lange.

Hadzic, A., & Vloka, J. (2004). Peripheral Nerve Blocks: Principles and Practice. New York: McGraw Hill.

Jensen, N. (2004). Big Yeller: Pain Killer for Boards. Iowa City: Anesthesia Board PREP. Web site: www.boardprep.com

Melzack, R., & Wall, P. (2005). Handbook of Pain Management. Philadelphia: Churchill Livingstone.

Netter, F. (1997). Atlas of Human Anatomy. East Hanover: Novartis.

O'Brien, M. (2000). Aids to the Examination of the Peripheral Nervous System. Philadelphia: Saunders.

Pappagallo, M., & Werner, M. (2008). Chronic Pain: A Primer for Physicians. Chicago: Remedica.

Pauwels, L., Akesson, E., & Stewart, P. (1988). Cranial Nerves. Philadelphia: B.C. Decker.

Raj, P., Lou, L., Erdine, S., Staats, P., & Waldman, S. (2003). Radiographic Imaging for Regional Anesthesia and Pain Management. Philadelphia: Churchill Livingstone.

Waldman, S. (2001). Interventional Pain Management. Philadelphia: Saunders.

Waldman, S. (2004). Atlas of Interventional Pain Management. Philadelphia: Saunders.

Index

N

Narcotic Scheduling, 146
Nerve Conduction Velocity, 80
Nerve injury, 166
Neurolysis
   Chemical Neurolysis, 66
   Subarachnoid, 67
Neuroma, 32, 76
Neuropathic Pain, 40, 45
   Deafferentation, 74
   Loss of segmental inhibition, 75, 76
Nicotinic receptors, 21
NMDA, 127, 139
Nociceptive Pain, 45
Nucleus pulposus, 12

O

Opiates
   Morphine, 144
Opioids
   Narcotic Scheduling, 146
   Partial antagonists, 143
   Reversal
      Naloxone, 146
Osgood-Schlatter disease, 113
Osteoarthritis, 104
Oswestry Disability Index, 53
Oucher scale, 111
Oxcarbazepine, 130
Oxycodone, 56, 145, 146

P

Pain Catastrophizing Scale, 157
Pain Disability Index, 53
Pancoast Tumor, 37
Paraneoplastic syndromes, 37
Parasympathetic nervous system, 20
Parkinson's Disease, 59, 102
Pelvic plexus. *See* Inferior Hypogastric Plexus
Periaqueductal Gray, 4, 5
Personality Disorders, 152
Phalen's sign, 24
Phantom limb pain, 77
Phenol. *See* Neurolysis
Phenytoin, 95, 98, 130, 132, 133
PLA-2, 89
Polymodal fibers. *See* C fibers
Polymyalgia Rheumatica, 51, 58, 105

Poly-Neuropathy, 78
Post Dural Puncture Headache, 172
Post Herpetic Neuralgia, 58
Postsynaptic Dorsal Column tract, 4
Pregabalin, 130
Pregnancy
   Anticonvulsants, 95
   Antidepressants, 96
   Aspirin and NSAIDs, 94
   Benzodiazepines, 96
   FDA classification of Drugs, 94
   Indomethacin use, 95
   Lactation and Medication, 97
   Migraine Medication, 96
   Opioids, 96
   Steroids, 96
Presacral Neurectomy, 121
Prialt, 84
Pudendal Nerve, 92, 93, 118

Q

Quantitative Sudomotor Axon Reflex Test, 81

R

Radiculitis, 16
Radiculopathy, 16
Radiofrequency Lesioning, 68
Ramsey-Hunt Syndrome, 51, 75
Raynaud's, 103
Rehabilitation modalities
   Cold Laser therapy, 169
Reiter's Syndrome, 105
Rheumatoid Arthritis, 57, 104
   Juvenile, 113

S

Sacral Plexus, 117
Samter's syndrome, 139
Scheuermann's disease, 113
Schmorl's node, 87
Sciatic nerve block, 165
SF 36, 53
Short Form McGill Pain Questionnaire, 55
Sickle Cell, 103
Somatoform Disorders, 154
Spina Bifida Occulta, 110
Spinal Cord Stimulation, 84
Spinal Stenosis, 14, 42

2912824